HANDS
ON

HANDS ON

Basic Clinical Skills for
Students and Practitioners
of Complementary and
Alternative Medicine

Nic Rowley

First published in 1994 by Hodder & Stoughton.

This edition published in 2018 by

Aeon Books Ltd
12 New College Parade
Finchley Road
London NW3 5EP

British Library Cataloguing in Publication Data

A C.I.P. for this book is available from the British Library

ISBN-13: 978-1-91159-730-8

This book is dedicated to my wife, Kirsten Hartvig.

CONTENTS

PREFACE

As accreditation standards become more stringent, the student of complementary medicine is coming under increasing pressure to acquire orthodox clinical examination skills as an aid to safe clinical decision making.

Eliciting clinical signs is a subtle art and cannot be learnt from books alone. Moreover, many of the techniques used by doctors are only relevant to a medical system that has become dependent on high tech, invasive investigations.

However, the basic clinical skills of listening, looking and feeling are common to all the healing arts. Hands on seeks to enhance and illuminate these skills in a way that is relevant to the needs of the complementary practitioner. As a consequence, some of the detail to be found in orthodox textbooks is omitted but it is hoped that readers will seek to broaden their knowledge through practical experience and by reference to standard texts.

I owe a debt of gratitude to many students and practitioners for their advice and support in the completion of this book and I would like to thank Dr Caroline Aldous, Dr Mike Robinson, Dr Richard James, Joe Nasr, Frances Kelly and Sai Baba for their particular help and inspiration.

ACKNOWLEDGEMENTS

The author and publishers would like to thank the following people for modelling in the book: Donna Andrews, Marjorie Boussemart, Timothy Corbishley, Marcus Ferreira, Elizabeth Gower, Lucinda Johnston, Kirsten Nottrot, Philippe Raoux, Bruce Smith and Helen Smith.

INTRODUCTION

There is no right way to take a history and examine a patient.

This book aims to demonstrate one way of approaching the task that you can adapt to your personal style and needs.

It is written in the belief that students of complementary medicine are presented with so much detailed information when first introduced to history taking and clinical examination that they never really understand why they are doing what they are doing.

The objectives of the book are therefore very simple:

1   To provide you with a basic set of questions to ask.
2   To teach you where to put your hands when examining a patient.

Your aims should be:

1   To develop a consistent clinical routine.
2   To practise this routine until you no longer have to think about what you are doing (or what you are supposed to do next).
3   To examine so many normal people that you will never fear missing the abnormal.
4   To be confident enough of your technique to allow you to perceive what your eyes, ears and hands are telling you.
5   To always be mindful of your client's comfort and dignity.
6   To be kind and gentle.
7   To explain to your client what you are doing.
8   To understand yourself why you are doing it.
9   To use the information you obtain to the benefit of your client.
10 To make decisions on the basis of your findings.

Clinical students are told from day one that the correct order for examining the patient is

LOOK

FEEL

TAP

LISTEN WITH THE STETHOSCOPE

or, in posh jargon,

OBSERVE

PALPATE

PERCUSS

AUSCULTATE

This routine is based on sound principles and it serves as a reminder that simply listening to what the patient has to say and observing him/her closely is usually all you have to do to gain the information necessary to formulate a relevant list of diagnostic possibilities.

In other words, much of what this book describes is likely to be unnecessary in most cases. However, someone once said that the trouble with life is that it has to be lived forwards but it can only be understood in reverse, and so it is with clinical examination. You only know it was unnecessary after you have done it.

In the orthodox medical model, history taking and clinical examination are supposed to generate a **differential diagnosis** (a list of diagnostic possibilities) which is refined by various investigative procedures into a **definitive diagnosis.** The definitive diagnosis is supposed to imply a causal link between demonstrable organic pathology and a particular clinical presentation. Having established this link beyond all reasonable doubt, the orthodox doctor is then supposed to make a logical intervention at the cellular, tissue or organ level in order to eradicate the underlying pathology.

The orthodox medical model can thus be summarized as follows:

TAKE A HISTORY

EXAMINE THE PATIENT

FORMULATE A DIFFERENTIAL DIAGNOSIS

PERFORM BASIC INVESTIGATIONS (urine analysis, blood tests, x-rays)

PERFORM SPECIALIST INVESTIGATIONS

CONFIRM THE DIAGNOSIS

TREAT THE UNDERLYING PATHOLOGY

FOLLOW UP THE PATIENT

Logical and laudable as this scheme is, however, it is rarely followed in practice due to the unswerving ability of patients to enliven their pathologies with mind, spirit, emotion, family and friends. Furthermore, without access to many of the investigations performed routinely by orthodox doctors, complementary practitioners often feel that it is irrelevant to perform an orthodox clinical assessment.

But, I believe that this misses the point which is that basic history taking and clinical examination is usually all you need to do to confirm that someone is WELL.

Never underestimate the importance of confirming wellness to your client – medical students are always lamenting the lack of 'real' pathology in their clinical experience. I think the best outcome of a medical encounter is one in which the patient is told that they are not a patient at all, i.e. that they are fit and well.

If you accept this, then you do not need to see a lot of pathology in your training. You need to see a lot of well people.

Some general thoughts:

- The range of normality is very wide indeed.
- Most *significant* clinical signs are as obvious as barn doors swinging in the wind.
- If you have not got a pretty good idea what is wrong with someone by the time they get on to your examination couch, you are unlikely to know what is wrong with them by the time they get off it.
- You are examining patients for their benefit and not to prove that you can perform the exercise in a technically correct manner.
- First clinical impressions are often the most accurate.
- Isolated clinical signs in obviously healthy people almost never suggest serious underlying pathology. Clinical signs only achieve significance in the context of the case history as a whole.

It is more important to be alert to warning symptoms and signs suggesting someone is seriously ill (and should thus be referred to expert help) than to understand the precise nature of the underlying problem. For example, the important things to notice in a patient with severe aortic stenosis are that they complain of angina, dizzy spells and shortness of breath on exertion and have a low volume pulse and a heart murmur. Describing the finer points of the murmur itself is not particularly important. Such a patient is ill and needs help. Basic history taking and examination are enough to demonstrate this.

PART I

HISTORY TAKING

1.1 APPROACHING THE PATIENT

First attempts at history taking are often thwarted by the desperate effort to remember what questions to ask in what order. Every practitioner knows the sinking feeling engendered by a blank mind (something which Zen aspirants may take years to achieve...); and yet an experienced practitioner often seems able to elicit reams of relevant information whilst hardly seeming to ask any questions at all.

This is not as difficult to do as it may seem.

The first trick is to understand what you are really trying to find out, i.e.:

- What has happened?
- To what kind of person?
- Why are they asking for help now?
- How is the problem affecting the person and their family?
- What sort of physical and social environment does the person come from?
- Do any of the complaints suggest the diagnosis of a 'disease'?

The second trick is not to ask too many questions. Let your client tell their own story in their own way.

The third trick is to conduct the interview in the same way as you would carry on a conversation with someone you know well. After all, twenty minutes history taking usually elucidates more private and personal information from a complete stranger than you probably know about your best friend.

The fourth trick – and this is by far the most important – is to be *interested* in your client. If you are really interested in what they are telling you and genuinely want to know how it happened and how it is affecting them, you will have no difficulty at all in remembering their story and filling in any gaps with a few well-chosen questions.

History taking presents a wonderful opportunity to establish a good relationship between you and a person looking for help and advice. Do not mess it up by assuming some sort of 'professional practitioner persona'; remember you only have one chance to make a first impression.

So, is there anything about your general approach to a patient that is likely to facilitate rather than hinder the process just described?

Well, first of all, I believe it is important to greet your client as an equal, giving them your full attention and performing whatever social rituals (shaking hands, etc) you feel comfortable with as a genuine expression of greeting.

It is then important to spend at least a couple of minutes in general, non-medical conversation to establish common ground and areas of mutual interest. You may find it convenient to ask the patient to fill in a simple data sheet listing name, address, job, etc, before the consultation starts. Reading this prior to meeting your client can help focus your attention and often provides a topic for some general chat. More importantly, it allows you to leave the pen on the desk and look the person in the eyes for the first few minutes of conversation.

When you start taking the structured history, make sure that the questions you use are in plain, unambiguous, colloquial language and that they are framed in such a way as to encourage your client to talk.

Try to avoid 'why' questions (why did you do that?) which tend to make people feel that they are being put on the spot to provide a right answer rather than a true one. Think of yourself as a good natured sheep dog – sometimes lying in the grass in the right spot is all that is needed to achieve results.

Above all, keep your questions open. Do not say 'you haven't got any pain there, have you?' because most people, being anxious to please and assuming that you must know anyway because you are medical, will simply agree with you.

Finally, keep paying attention. Do not worry about writing things down; if you are really interested, you will remember what is important when you come to write a concise summary later on. Look at the person talking to you as much as possible and you will be amazed at how much you are learning about their problem. Avoid asking questions twice. This will reduce the risk of your patient thinking that you are yet another practitioner who seems to come from a different reality from the rest of humankind.

1.2 THE QUESTIONS TO ASK

Traditionally, a case history is elucidated in more or less the following order (acronyms commonly used as case note headings are given in brackets):

- The patient's complaint (c/o – means 'complaining of')
- The history of the presenting problem (HPP)
- The past medical history (PMH)
- Drug history, including details of immunizations
- History of illness in the family (FH)
- Social history (SH)
- Dietary history
- A systematic enquiry into the general health of the patient at the time of the consultation (SQ)

I will go on to list all the various questions to be asked under each heading and have also summarized them at the end of the book (Part 4.2).

In order to learn quickly, you first have to accept the fact that, for the first two or three months, you will forget to ask lots of important things. But, after all, you are supposed to be learning so it does not matter; it is your supervisors' responsibility to make sure that each case is appropriately managed.

Having accepted this, I suggest that the only list you have on your desk for your first twenty or thirty cases is the list of headings given above. *Talk* to the patient about each subject area, find out what you can and do not write anything down (really) until you have heard the whole story. If nothing else, this will avoid a lot of crossing out and starting again.

Afterwards, you can compare the story you obtained with the full list of questions given overleaf and see what you have left out. More important, you can check whether you have left out anything significant. If you have, resolve to remember to get the information at the next consultation.

Bit by bit, week by week, you will find that you are asking the relevant questions by instinct and, what is more, you will have got into the habit of talking to, and looking at, your clients. You will also be working more quickly than many of your colleagues since you won't be wasting time writing things down until you are sure that what you are writing down is relevant.

The *systematic enquiry* (SQ) is the cause of much grief to students, patients and teachers alike and often takes up a disproportionate amount of the interview time. This is to misunderstand its function, which is to review, briefly and rapidly, those aspects of the patient's health which have not been covered in the history of the presenting complaint. If you have heard everything about your client's heart or chest (or whatever) during the HPP, do not ask it all over again in the SQ. You know it already.

Conversely, if a client starts off by telling you things that suggest problems with the heart or chest, make sure you ask all the relevant SQ questions on heart and chest during the HPP. It will also save you time if you remember that the SQ is not supposed to gather information about the past; that should have been done under the heading 'Past Medical History'.

In other words, the purpose of the SQ is to give you the chance to ask the patient whether they are suffering today from any complaints which they might have neglected to mention but which might, to you, be relevant.

Cut down to its bare essentials, therefore, taking a history can be reduced to the following simple questions:

- How can I help you? (a good opening gambit this; less restricting than 'what seems to be the problem?' It may turn out that they do not, in fact, have a problem and, more important, it establishes the idea that you are there to help rather than to 'treat'. It is sometimes enough to draw out a complete HPP)
- When did you last feel completely well? (i.e. is today's problem just one more damn thing after another or is it something new and out of context with the rest of your life)
- Have you been generally well in the past? (leads to a discussion of PMH)
- Are you taking any medication or supplements of any kind at the moment? (leads into drug history)
- Do you come from a healthy family? (leads into FH)
- How are things at work? (SH)
- How are things at home? (SH)
- Do you smoke? (SH)
- Do you drink alcohol? (SH)
- Do you take much exercise? (SH)
- What's your diet like?

In this rudimentary scheme, and in practice when time is short, the essentials of a SQ can be elicited by the following questions:

- Do you have a fever at the moment ?
- Do you have any skin rash?
- Do you get short of breath?
- Do you have a cough?
- Do you have any chest pain?
- Are your bowels OK?
- How is your appetite?
- How is your weight?
- Are your waterworks OK?
- Do you get headaches?
- Do you get dizzy spells?
- Are you sleeping OK?

Hippocrates said *'it is more important to know what sort of person has a disease than what sort of disease a person has'*. This is more than a plea for holism: it is a vitally important aspect of clinical information gathering. Formulating an appropriate differential diagnosis depends on understanding the context of a person's problem (babies rarely get cancer, old people rarely get whooping cough) and if your history taking allows you to answer only the few questions listed above, you are more likely to be able to understand what is wrong than the student who has slavishly filled in six pages of detailed history sheet.

Having, hopefully, encouraged you to practise history taking with the aid of minimal lists and even more minimal note taking, I will now list the components of a full, formal case history under standard headings.

Remember, however, that this is not necessarily the order in which you will write things down when recording the history in the case notes (see Part 1.3 and Part 2).

Case History

Personal Details
Date of Birth
Sex
Name
Address
Telephone numbers
Occupation
Marital status
Children
General practitioner details
Route of referral or recommendation
Previous experience of complementary medicine
Date of first consultation

Presenting Problem(s)
Keep this as succinct as possible
One or two lines is enough
Try to record the patient's actual words

History of Presenting Problem
When were they last completely well?
When did it start?
What was happening at the time?
Did it start suddenly or gradually?
How has it progressed?
What brings it on?
What makes it worse?
What makes it better?
Are there any associated problems?
Have they had it before and, if yes, what diagnostic tests and treatments have they had for it?

If somebody complains of pain, remember also to ask about:
- The site of the pain
- Its quality (sharp or dull)
- Whether it is localized or diffused

- Whether it is intermittent or continuous
- Whether it moves or has moved position
- Whether any other symptoms accompany the pain

Past Medical History

Any childhood diseases
Any serious illnesses
Any accidents
Any admissions to hospital
Any operations
Obstetric history if female

Also ask specifically about:
- Hepatitis/jaundice (may be Hepatitis B carrier)
- Rheumatic fever (rheumatic fever in early life predisposes to valvular heart disease later on. St Vitus' dance and acute glomerulonephritis are also associated with rheumatic fever)
- Diabetes
- TB
- Glandular fever
- Sexually transmitted diseases
- Asthma, hay fever, eczema (may suggest allergic tendency)

Drug History

Name of each drug
Taken for what
Dosage and frequency of administration
How long taken for

Ask specifically about:
- Laxatives
- Antacids
- Sleeping pills
- Oral contraceptives
- Vitamins
- Minerals
- Homoeopathic remedies
- Herbal remedies
- Vaccinations

Allergies
Any known allergies (including to drugs)

Family History
Enquire about the health of:
- Mother
- Father
- Sisters and brothers

Also, find out if there is any family tendency to particular diseases (especially heart disease, high blood pressure, stroke and diabetes) and if there are any known inherited diseases in the family

Social History
Get a picture of the home situation
Get a picture of the work situation

Discuss:
- Exercise
- Smoking
- Drinking
- Recreational drugs
- Relationships
- Sex

Diet
Build up a picture of an average week's eating and drinking

Systematic Enquiry
Remember, do not ask questions to which you already know the answer.

Also remember that you are asking about how they are today, not how they were five years ago.

If something significant comes up, ask general questions about onset, progression, aggravating factors and relieving factors as for the history of the presenting complaint.

Sometimes, pressure of time may dictate that you do not follow up additional complaints revealed in the SQ until a later consultation.

Cardiovascular system
Ask about
Chest pain
Shortness of breath on exertion
Shortness of breath when lying flat (orthopnoea)
Palpitations
Swelling of the ankles (ankle oedema)
Varicose veins
Cold hands or feet

Respiratory system
As for heart plus ask about
Catarrh
Earache
Sore throat
Cough
Sputum production
Coughing up blood (haemoptysis)
Wheezing

Gastro-intestinal tract
Ask about
Appetite
Weight change
Dental problems
Nausea
Indigestion
Problems swallowing
Vomiting
Abdominal pain
Vomiting blood (haematemesis)
Flatulence
Diarrhoea/constipation
Unusual looking faeces (bloody, very pale, very dark)
Rectal bleeding

Urinary tract
Ask about
Urgency (having to go very badly, very suddenly)
Frequency (having to go often)
Dysuria (hurting or burning when you go)
Haematuria (blood in the urine)
Loin pain (because that is where your kidneys are)
Difficulty starting urination
Poor stream of urine
Difficulty stopping urination (dribbling, incontinence)
Unusually smelly, frothy or discoloured urine

Nervous system
Ask about
Poor sleep
Headaches
Disturbance of vision
Loss of hearing
Tinnitus (ringing in the ears)
Dizziness or vertigo (vertigo is the sensation of the world moving around you when you are stationary)
Fainting
Fits
Muscle weakness
Pins and needles or other odd sensations
Mood swings
Disturbances of memory or concentration

Endocrine system
Ask about
Intolerance of heat
Intolerance of cold
Polyuria (large volume of urine passed often)
Polydipsia (drinking a lot of fluid)

Musculoskeletal system

Ask about

Joint pain

Joint stiffness

Joint swelling

Backache

Skin

Ask about

Skin rashes

Lumps or bumps

Unusual moles

Reproductive system

Ask about

Sexual problems (the question 'are you happy with the sexual side of the relationship with your partner' rarely causes embarrassment)

Sexually transmitted diseases (may be complaints of urethral discharge, genital irritation or sores)

Contraception

Infertility

Impotence

For women

Age periods started (menarche)

Length of cycle (from day one of period to day one of the next period)

Are periods regular?

How heavy?

How painful?

Any distressing premenstrual symptoms?

Any bleeding between periods?

Any vaginal discharge?

Painful intercourse?

How many times pregnant?

Discuss pregnancies and births in detail

Any miscarriages?

Any abortions?

Where appropriate, age periods stopped and any problems associated with the climacteric/menopause

1.3 RECORDING INFORMATION

Writing detailed notes during the taking of a case history can cause problems:

- It takes too long. Both you and the patient have a limited concentration span and the quality of your note taking by the end of the consultation will be diminished if you keep pausing to write.
- It interferes with the flow of conversation and obstructs the development of rapport between you and your client.
- You are likely to write things down that have to be changed as the story unfolds and your client relaxes.
- You will end up with notes so detailed and dense that nobody (including you) can be bothered to read them properly in the future.

Clinical notes should, on subsequent reading, bring a picture of that particular patient immediately to mind. There is thus a need to condense the information gained into a succinct form.

I therefore recommend that you:

- Carefully record basic personal details at the top of your case history sheet.
- Jot down only key words, figures and phrases on a piece of scrap paper during the history telling.
- Write the relevant information, in summary form, on to a pre-prepared case history sheet (see example in Part 3.8) whilst the patient is getting ready to be examined, or even after the consultation is over.
- Go through your physical examination routine without taking notes (apart from jotting down any particular measurements like blood pressure) and, again, record the information on a pre-prepared sheet as your patient is getting dressed.
- Do not institute a plan of management without committing your assessment of the case to paper (this usually involves some statement of differential diagnosis).
- When the consultation is over, spend just a couple of minutes writing a four or five line summary of the case and constructing a problem list (see below). The time spent will be amply rewarded in the next consultation when the facts of the case are brought instantly to mind by a glance at the summary.

The following tips will help you to avoid infuriating and embarrassing omissions in your case notes:

- Take your time writing down personal details at the beginning of the consultation. The epidemiological data they contain form the foundation of your clinical assessment.
- Write the date of the consultation (and every subsequent consultation) at the start of the notes.
- As far as possible, write down fact rather than conjecture. If the use of medical jargon commits you to a concept or diagnosis that you do not truly believe, write down what you really do know in plain English. (Put another way, it can be very frustrating to start a consultation with a complaint of 'headache' only to find, after 45 minutes, that history taking and examination have left you no further on than knowing that your client has a headache. Nevertheless, if that is the situation, it is better to acknowledge it and deal with the problem as best you can rather than try to treat a non-existent 'disease'.)
- Don't sit on the fence. Commit yourself. Write down what you have found, not what other people are said to have found. If you are not sure whether you have found something or not, you probably have not. Do not write things down like: 'Bit of an aortic murmur' or 'reflexes perhaps a bit reduced on the left'. In terms of patient management, symptoms and signs are either there or they are not. In other words, BELIEVE WHAT YOU PERCEIVE AND ACT ACCORDINGLY.
- Always take the time to record full details of your client's current medication.
- Always construct a management plan (see page 15) and record exactly what you have advised your patient to do. It is sometimes helpful to keep a duplicate of any written advice or instructions that you may give.

Recording the Results of a Clinical Examination

The order in which clinical examination is performed is not the same as the order in which examination findings are usually recorded. The standard formats for each system are given in Part Two and are summarized at the end of the book.

Summaries

The case summary is the key to your clinical assessment. It forces you to marshal your thoughts and write down only what you think is really important. It provides a clear *aide mémoire* for subsequent consultations and it forms the basis of any letters you may write to other practitioners, etc.

Always start a case summary with a thumbnail sketch of the person concerned and then mention only the significant positive and negative clinical findings. For example:

A 55 year old married bus driver smoking 40 cigarettes per day since age 15 yrs. Complaining of a six month history of central crushing chest pain brought on by minimal exertion (such as climbing stairs) and relieved by 10 minutes rest. There is a family history of sudden cardiac death and hypercholesterolaemia. Examination of the cardiovascular system revealed a blood pressure of 165/100. The fundi were normal and there were no other abnormal clinical findings.

Problem Lists

A problem list is simply a piece of paper on which all the problems revealed in the history are listed under one of the following headings:

Active (i.e. causing difficulty now)

Inactive (i.e. not causing immediate difficulty but providing a context for your patient's other complaints)

Each problem entry is dated as it is written.

The beauty of problem lists is that they enable you to judge at a glance how your patient is progressing from week to week. However much therapy you may have thrown at them, if the problem list at the end of your course of treatment is (from the patient's point of view) no different than when they first met you, you have not really helped them much.

Problem lists should take as much account of emotional, intellectual and spiritual problems as of physical problems. Resolving the former often has a profound effect on the latter.

Management Plans

A decent management plan is more than just a list of remedies, treatments or manipulations. It should state:

- What further investigations are needed (if any), when and by whom.
- Explanations you have given to your client explaining their current state of health and the principles behind any treatment offered.
- Any dietary, lifestyle or other general advice.
- Clear, specific descriptions of remedies, treatments, manipulations, etc. If a remedy of any kind is being supplied, remember to state how often and in what way it is to be taken, whether any food, drink or other medication is to be avoided and how many days or weeks the treatment is supposed to continue.
- The date of the next consultation and any other follow-up arrangements.

Follow-up Records

I suggest that notes for follow-up consultations are recorded under four headings.

- Subjective (what the patient tells you)
- Objective (what you observe)
- Assessment (what do you think is going on. Have things got better, worse or stayed the same)
- Plan (what are you going to do about it)

The benefits of this system (called SOAP for short) are enormous and are a major protection against dangerous conjecture, misunderstanding and indecision.

Conclusion

The system just outlined produces what is known as a Problem Oriented Medical Record (POMR).

A POMR has four parts:

A database made up from the information collected during history taking and examination.

2 A problem list.

3 A management plan.

4 Follow-up notes.

Whilst this scheme is not as elaborate as that used by some orthodox institutions, it retains the central characteristic of being *patient-oriented*. In other words, it ensures that you are aware of how things are affecting the patient at all times and encourages you to adopt broad based management strategies based on your client's actual problems rather than your diagnoses.

1.4 CASE TAKING IN PSYCHOLOGICAL MEDICINE

Assessing whether someone is mentally ill or not is one of the hardest tasks in medicine and it is probably fair to say that even orthodox psychiatrists find the conventional medical model inappropriate to the task. There is much argument about what constitutes mental illness and psychiatrists work extremely hard to maintain a consensus on which disturbances of thought, emotion and behaviour constitute psychiatric morbidity. They have thus developed a precise but complex language to describe the phenomena they observe, some of which is explained at the end of this section.

Many orthodox doctors would say that no 'unqualified' person should become involved in the management of mental disturbance but it is a fact that many people labelled 'mentally ill' are drawn to investigate alternative and complementary medical disciplines, hoping to find a refuge from drug based management.

I believe it is important, therefore, for you to have a method of clinical assessment that is likely to

1   alert you to the possibility that a client may be mentally unwell;
2   allow you to make a basic assessment of the seriousness of the situation so that appropriate referral can be made if necessary;
3   alert you to the presence of **organic brain dysfunction** (physical brain disease) so that treatable pathologies are not overlooked;
4   protect you from preconception and bias in your dealings with the mentally ill.

This section will outline questions of particular relevance to a psychiatric case history and will define a number of common terms used in the description of mental illness.

The mental equivalent of physical examination, the **Mental State Examination**, is described in Part 2.6.

Note: It can be very helpful to obtain third party corroboration of information obtained during a psychiatric case history from a relative or friend of the client.

The Psychiatric Case History

Personal Details
As for ordinary case history (see page 6)

Presenting Problem(s)
As for ordinary case history but often hard to define

Factual Personal History
Birth date
Birth place
Birth difficulties
Age walking
Age talking
Age dry at night
Age toilet trained
School record (including exams)
Higher education record if appropriate
Jobs: where, how many, how long,
Sexual relationships: first experiences, how many
Marriage/partnership: Date, partner age, job, etc
Children: how many, when born

Present Circumstances
Marriage/partnership: how is it going?
Job: where, how is it going?
Housing: where, what is it like?
Finances: any current problems?
Hobbies: what are they, how often done?
Friends: how many, how close?

Family History
As for ordinary case history but remember to ask specifically about family history of mental illness

Past Medical and Psychiatric History
As for normal case history but remember to ask about previous episodes of mental illness and their management, suicide attempts, etc

Drugs and Allergies
As for ordinary case history

Habits
Smoking, drinking, recreational drugs, criminal activity, brushes with the law

Personality
Ask your client to give a picture of their personality both through their own eyes and through those of their family and friends

General Medical History
Take a brief general medical history if possible. This information may be crucial in confirming or excluding organic pathology as a cause of the mental problems

The Language of Psychiatry

The following list of definitions is not exhaustive and is meant solely as an introduction to a complex subject.

Anorexia nervosa
Persistent, active refusal to eat accompanied by profound weight loss and physiological disturbance.

Cyclothymia
Marked mood swings between elation and depression.

Delirium
An extreme state of organic brain dysfunction characterized by disorientation, illusions, hallucinations, overactivity and altered levels of consciousness. Delirium Tremens (DTs) is the acute organic brain syndrome provoked by withdrawal from alcohol and some drugs.

Delusion
A fixed, firm, false belief, inappropriate to a person's ethnic, social or religious background and held in the face of logical argument. Delusions are important symptoms of psychosis and take many forms including:

- Interference with thoughts
- Being controlled
- Paranoia
- Guilt
- Grandiosity
- Nihilism
- Misinterpretation
- Hypochondriasis
- Religious significance
- Ideas of reference in which the sufferer believes that newspaper articles, TV and radio broadcasts, etc, all refer to him/her

Depersonalization
Feeling unreal, not one's self.

Derealization
The feeling that the world around is strange or dreamlike.

Endogenous (psychotic) depression
Profound depression complicated by delusions (often of guilt or hypochondriasis) with associated disturbance of bowel habit, appetite and sleep.

Flight of ideas
A way of talking in which the speaker moves from one topic to another at an alarming rate. Rhymes, puns or loose association of ideas may trigger off the changes of topic.

Hallucination
A sensory perception that occurs without an obvious external stimulus.

Hypomania
A state of extreme overactivity, elation and excitement (sometimes accompanied by hallucinations and/or delusions).

Illusion

A *misinterpretation* of a sensory perception (such as thinking that the policeman coming towards you is a monster with two heads and red eyes (unless, of course...)).

Neurosis

Psychiatric illness (including non-psychotic depression, anxiety states, obsessional and phobic disorders) in which contact with reality is maintained (i.e. no hallucinations or delusions).

Organic Brain Syndrome

Physical damage to brain tissue affects **cognitive** ability, i.e. it causes disturbances of consciousness, memory and orientation in time and space (who am I, where am I). The major chronic organic brain syndrome is dementia. Fever, poisoning, drugs and lack of oxygen may cause acute organic brain disorder.

Paranoia

Paranoia means 'beyond reason' and is thus used by psychiatrists to describe the features of psychosis. It covers more than the colloquial concept of persecution and includes feelings of grandeur, jealousy, love, envy, hate, the supernatural, etc.

Psychosis

A disturbance of thought, emotion and volition severe enough to distort awareness of the world. A 'breakdown in reality testing'.

Psychosomatic

The influence of mental function on body function.

Psychopathic

Seriously irresponsible, antisocial, immature and impulsive behaviour combined with an inability to tolerate frustration. May lead to aggression or an inadequate state in which normal duties and responsibilities are neglected.

Schizophrenia
A psychotic condition characterized by disordered thought and delusions.

Stereotypies
Repetitive, voluntary movement patterns not explained by a neurological disorder (e.g. head banging).

Tics
Rapid, involuntary, repetitive, purposeless movements not caused by a neurological disorder.

1.5 SIGNIFICANT FINDINGS IN THE CASE HISTORY

Complementary medical students are often faced with a paradox:

Their teachers tell them it is desirable to perform detailed physical examinations on all patients but admit that they rarely do so themselves in their own practices.

It is, therefore, very hard for students to develop a feel for what constitutes good grounds for performing a clinical examination in the 'real life' practice situation. Things are further complicated by the fact that physical examination is often taught in such exhaustive detail that there never seems to be enough time to examine patients properly in the teaching clinic. Because of this, many students never examine at all when they finally qualify and start in practice.

I believe that this is at best a great shame and at worst dangerous. I contend that it is quite possible for all practitioners to learn quick, basic clinical examination routines and that these should always be performed in full. Listening to the heart, for example, without having felt the pulse, taken the blood pressure, located the apex beat, etc, will produce no useful information since individual clinical signs have to be woven into a pattern on the cloth of the case history before sensible diagnostic deductions can be made. No physical sign can be interpreted in isolation.

On the other hand, I must acknowledge that there are many situations in which performing clinical examination is probably unnecessary or irrelevant (when were you last examined by your general practitioner?).

One resolution to this dilemma is to examine quickly those systems that relate to complaints mentioned in the HPP. Thus if a patient complains of breathlessness, examine the cardiovascular and respiratory systems. If they complain of rectal bleeding, examine the gastro-intestinal system in full (including a rectal examination). Family history of disease also merits relevant clinical examination (e.g. you should examine the cardiovascular system of people with a family history of sudden cardiac death).

The object of the next part of the book is to convince you that the various body systems can be examined quickly and reliably in about five minutes each. This will, hopefully, encourage you to use the routines described whenever case history findings suggest the need for clinical examination.

PART 2

BASIC EXAMINATION
PROCEDURES

INTRODUCTION

Hands on aims to help you get the most out of your practical clinical training by encouraging you to develop quick, logical and useable clinical examination routines.

Each of the following six sections starts with a brief summary of the examination routine for the system involved. This is followed by pages containing photographs of certain steps being applied in practice with hints and tips on how to perform the techniques illustrated. Each section ends with a summary of how the information obtained should be recorded in the notes.

The emphasis throughout is on the description of the various examination techniques. Information concerning the detailed interpretation of particular clinical findings should be sought in textbooks of general medicine.

However, I strongly suggest that you do not spend too much time reading about the significance of abnormal physical signs until you can perform the routines outlined in Part Two almost without thinking. Once your hands have learnt what to do, your mind will be released to think about *what* you are discovering. You will then be in a better position to consider the diagnostic significance of your findings.

Note that it is standard practice for a right-handed practitioner to stand on the patient's right-hand side when examining. There is no particularly convincing reason for this convention but it looks neat and allows you to concentrate on the patient's face (when necessary) without your examining arm getting in the way.

Also, at any time during the examination of any system, you may come across a lump, bump or swelling. These must be fully assessed and a full description of the appropriate method is given in Part 3.1.

2.1 EXAMINING THE CARDIOVASCULAR SYSTEM

Basic Routine

- Observe the general state of your patient
- Look at the hands
- Assess the radial pulses
- Take the blood pressure
- Assess the height of the jugular venous pulse (JVP)
- Feel the carotid pulses
- Look at the colour of the conjunctivae
- Look at the tongue and mucous membranes of the mouth
- Look at the praecordium (the part of the chest overlying the heart)
- Assess the position of the apex beat
- Feel the chest for heaves and thrills
- Listen to the heart at the apex with the diaphragm of your stethoscope
- Listen to the heart at the left sternal edge with the diaphragm of your stethoscope
- Listen to the heart in the second *right* intercostal space with the diaphragm of your stethoscope
- Listen to the heart in the second *left* intercostal space with the diaphragm of your stethoscope
- Listen to these four areas again using the bell of your stethoscope. When you listen at the apex with the bell, lean the patient over to the left slightly
- Sit the patient forward and listen at the left sternal edge with the diaphragm of your stethoscope, with the patient holding their breath in expiration
- Listen to the base of the lungs on the left and the right
- Feel over the sacrum for pitting oedema
- Lie the patient back and then try to find the dorsalis pedis and posterior tibial pulses in the feet
- Feel the ankles for pitting oedema
- Look at the fundi through an ophthalmoscope

STEP BY STEP

PROCEDURE:
Observe the general state of your patient

Hints and tips
Do not stand too close.

Try to form a general impression (how ill are they, are they anxious, sweating or in pain).

Look at the colour of the skin and mucous membranes (pale, cyanosed).

Observe the breathing (fast, laboured).

PROCEDURE:
Look at the hands

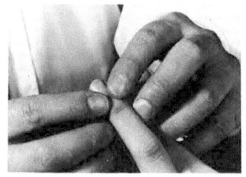 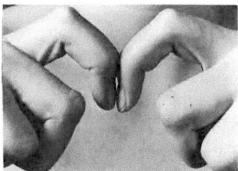

Figure 1a   Figure 1b

Hints and tips
Do the ends of the fingers look 'clubbed'? (Clubbing is swelling of the subcutaneous tissues over the terminal phalanges.)

If they do, feel the soft tissue at the base of each nail using the tips of your index fingers (Figure 1a) to assess fluctuance (squishyness). Clubbed fingers feel abnormally fluctuant. Then look to see if the angle at the base of any nail has been obliterated by subcutaneous swelling by asking the patient to hold the ends of their fingers together in front of you, nail to nail (Figure 1b), one pair after another. If you can not see a clear gap at the base of each pair of nails, the fingers may be clubbed.

Clubbing is an important sign that may accompany cyanotic congenital heart disease, bacterial endocarditis, serious chronic lung disease and some chronic gastro-intestinal conditions (e.g. cirrhosis of the liver and inflammatory bowel disease). However, some perfectly healthy people have congenitally clubbed fingers.

Is there any other evidence of heart disease? For example, are there any small 'splinter haemorrhages' under the nails (seen in normal people doing manual work and ill people with bacterial endocarditis) or painful red lumps (Osler's Nodes) in the finger pulps (another sign of infectious endocarditis).

Do the nails look blue (peripheral cyanosis) suggesting poor perfusion of the extremities?

PROCEDURE:
Assess the radial pulses (Figure 2)

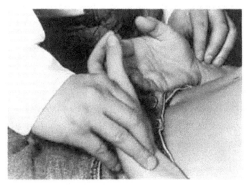

Figure 2

Hints and tips
Once you have decided that both radial pulses are present, concentrate on one.

Assess the rate (number of beats in 15 seconds × 4).

Is the rhythm regular or irregular (it is normal for the heart to speed up slightly on inspiration and slow down slightly on expiration)?

Is the pulse volume large or small?

Is there anything striking about the waveform of the pulse?

PROCEDURE:
Take the blood pressure

Hints and tips
This procedure is described in detail in Part 3.5.

PROCEDURE:
Assess the height of the jugular venous pulse (JVP)

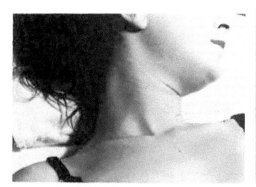 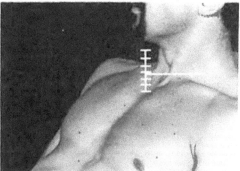

Figure 3a   Figure 3b

Hints and tips
Lie the patient at 45 degrees with their head relaxed on the pillows and turned away from you (Figure 3a). It will be easier to see the JVP if there is light coming from a window or lamp on the side opposite to you.

In a normal person lying at 45 degrees, the JVP can usually be seen between the heads of the sternomastoid (just above the clavicle) as a complex waveform that gets more prominent on inspiration.

However, it is sometimes quite difficult to see the JVP and, when you do see it, it is often difficult to distinguish it from the pulsation of the carotid artery. Remember that you can feel the carotid pulse but not the JVP.

Pulsation in the external jugular vein is often easier to see than pulsation in the internal jugular vein. Although anatomical variation makes the external jugular vein a less reliable indicator of the height of the JVP, many practitioners take the height of the pulsation in the external jugular vein to represent the height of the JVP.

The height of the JVP should be no more than about 3cm vertically above the manubrio-sternal angle (see Figure 3b to see how this is measured) but anxiety can cause some increase so do not be too quick to assume pathology in a patient with a slightly raised JVP who is obviously perfectly well.

Since the aim is to assess the height of the JVP, the important thing is to make sure that you have really seen the 'top' of the waveform.

The following methods are thus useful ways of checking the height of the JVP:

Suppose you can not see the JVP at all. Occlude the jugular veins by applying pressure with the edge of a finger to the root of the neck, just above the clavicle. See Figure 4.

The jugular veins (the external will be the obvious one) will fill up from above and become distended after about five seconds. Remove your finger. If the veins empty immediately and no complex pulsation remains visible, you can be fairly confident that the JVP is not raised.

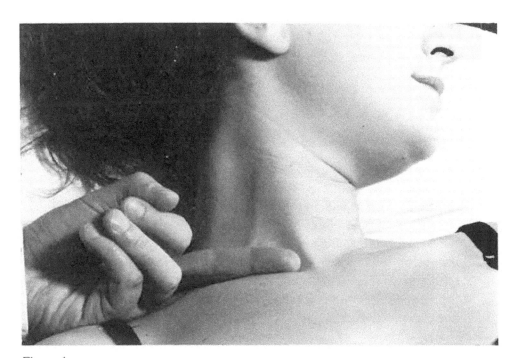

Figure 4

2   Alternatively, having occluded the veins at the root of the neck with the middle finger of your right hand, milk the blood upwards out of the external jugular vein with the middle finger of your left hand to just below the angle of the jaw. See Figure 5.

Keeping the upper finger in place, release the lower finger. If the JVP is raised, the vein will fill up from below to a height greater than 3cm above the manubrio-sternal angle.

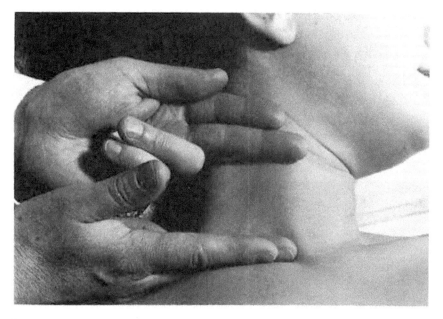

Figure 5

3   A more formal way of demonstrating the top of the JVP that is effective but slightly uncomfortable for the patient is to elicit the 'hepato-jugular reflex'. This simply means that if you press on the lower edge of the liver below the ribs with the flat of your hand, extra blood will be pushed back towards the heart, thus artificially and temporarily raising the JVP. Seeing the JVP move up and down as you do this reassures you that you really have seen the top of the waveform!

PROCEDURE:

Feel the carotid pulses (Figure 6)

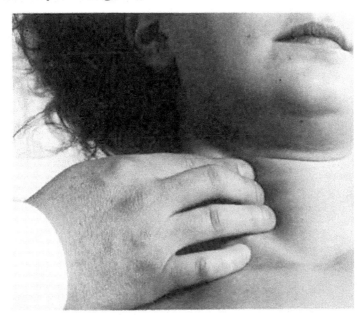

Figure 6

Hints and tips

It is not always necessary to feel the carotid pulses but most people find that it is easier to discern the waveform of a pulse in larger arteries (e.g. the carotid or the brachial).

If you do palpate the carotid pulse remember:

- Only feel one side at a time
- Don't press too hard (remember the carotid bodies)
- Some people dislike having their neck touched

PROCEDURE:
Look at the colour of the conjunctivae

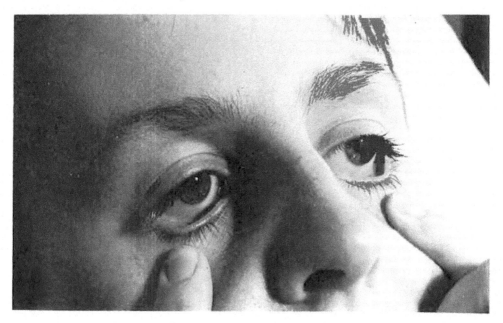

Figure 7

Hints and tips
It is less invasive to ask the patient to pull their own eyelids down whilst you examine the colour of the conjunctivae (see Figure 7). If they are unusually pale, the patient may be anaemic.

Look at each iris for an arcus senilis (a white line around the cornea) and also look around the eyes for xanthelasma (small yellow lumps of cholesterol under the skin). Arcus senilis is common in the elderly but suggests hyperlipidaemia if found in younger patients. Xanthelasma may also be associated with hyperlipidaemia.

PROCEDURE:
Look at the tongue and mucous membranes of the mouth

Hints and tips
Look for bluish discoloration suggesting central cyanosis.

PROCEDURE:
Look at the praecordium (the part of the chest overlying the heart)

Hints and tips
Are there any abnormal pulsations visible?

PROCEDURE:
Assess the position of the apex beat (Figure 8)

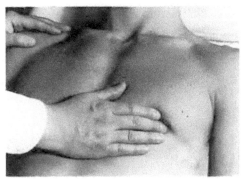
Figure 8

Hints and tips
The apex beat is normally found in the fifth left intercostal space (ICS) in the mid-clavicular line. This is not as far down the chest as you might think.

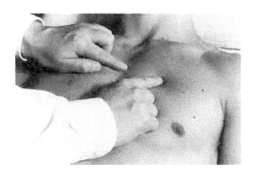
Figure 9

The best way to find the fifth ICS is to locate the second ICS (directly opposite the manubrio-sternal angle) (see Figure 9) and then count down to the fifth. If the apex beat seems displaced, try to determine the lowest and most lateral point at which the pulsation is distinctly felt.

As you feel the apex beat, try to assess its character.

Note that it can be difficult to find the apex beat in muscular and obese people. Leaning the patient over to the left (which brings the heart closer to the chest wall) sometimes helps.

PROCEDURE:
Feel the chest for heaves and thrills

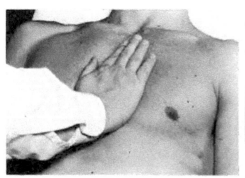

Figure 10a

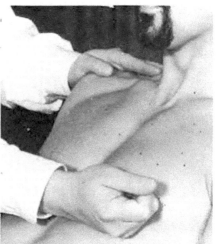

Figure 10b

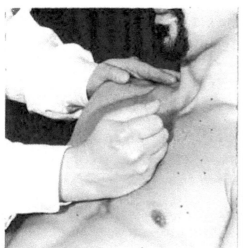

Figure 10c

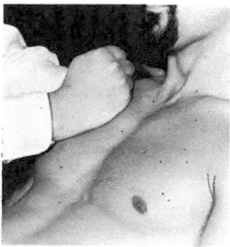

Figure 10d

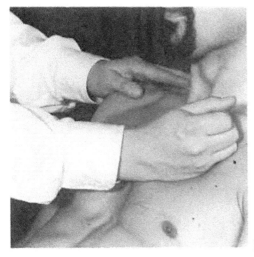

Figure 10e

Hints and tips

a) Lay your hand flat over the left edge of the sternum (Figure 10a). If the right ventricle is enlarged, the sternum will seem to rock up and down with each heart beat. This is known as a 'parasternal heave'.

b) Feel with the flat or edge of your hand over the apex (Figure 10b), at the left sternal edge (Figure 10c) and in second right ICS (Figure 10d), and second left ICS (Figure 10e). See if you can feel any 'thrills'. A thrill is a heart murmur so loud that you can feel it. Generations of medical students have been told that thrills feel similar to the sensation of holding a buzzing bluebottle in your hand, which is probably as good a way of describing them as any.

PROCEDURE:

a) Listen to the heart at the apex with the diaphragm of your stethoscope (Figure 11a)

b) Listen to the heart at the left sternal edge with the diaphragm of your stethoscope (Figure 11b)

c) Listen to the heart in the second right intercostal space with the diaphragm of your stethoscope (Figure 11c)

d) Listen to the heart in the second left intercostal space with the diaphragm of your stethoscope (Figure 11d)

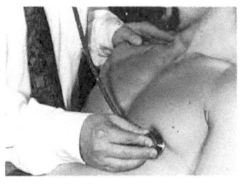

Figure 11a

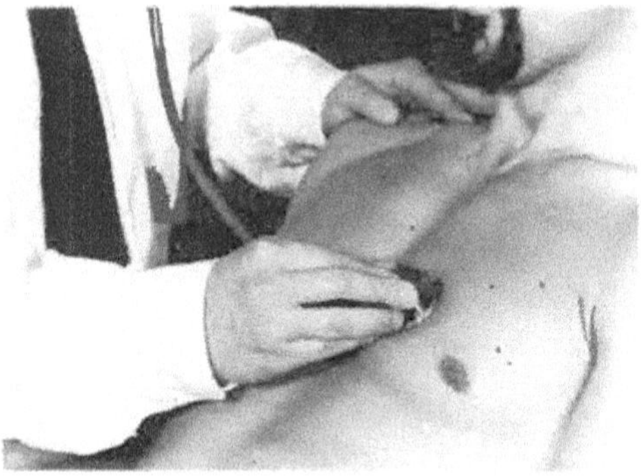

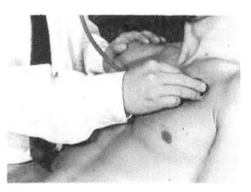

Figure 11b

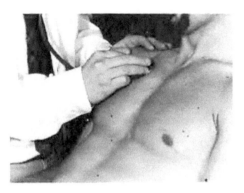

Figure 11c

Figure 11d

Hints and tips

It is not necessary to spend ages listening to the heart in each position; you merely have to listen long enough to:

- Hear the first and second heart sounds
- Hear any added (third or fourth) heart sounds that might be present
- See if you can hear any murmurs.

If you find it hard to distinguish between the first and second sounds (dummm-da, dummm-da dummm-da or, if you prefer, lub-dup, lub-dup, lub-dup), feel the carotid pulse gently as you listen. The pulse is felt immediately *after* the first heart sound.

If either the first or the second heart sounds appear to be 'double' (split), this is probably normal, especially in young people. The clarity of the split of a normal second sound diminishes as the patient breathes out.

The tricky thing is to distinguish between a *split* heart sound and an *added* heart sound.

It may help to remember that added heart sounds tend to be low pitched and are thus more clearly heard with the bell of the stethoscope.

Third heart sounds are heard after the second heart sound producing a dummm-dada, dummm-dada type of rhythm.

Fourth heart sounds occur just before the first heart sound and produce a dadumm-da, dadumm-da, dadumm-da sort of rhythm.

The significance of third and fourth heart sounds varies from patient to patient but, in healthy young people, they are unlikely to represent pathology.

In patients with left heart failure, the combination of an added heart sound and a fast pulse rate produces a sound with the rhythm of a cantering horse (referred to as a gallop rhythm).

Murmurs are reflections of heart valve dysfunction. They are heard as whooshing or blowing sounds filling in the gaps between the heart sounds. If you think you hear a murmur, you should try to work out the following:

- Does the murmur occur between the first and second heart sounds (in which case it is *systolic*) or after the second and before the first (in which case it is *diastolic*)?
- Is the murmur high-pitched or low-pitched?
- Is the murmur loud or soft?
- Where is it heard most distinctly; can it be heard in several areas (i.e. does the sound 'radiate' from the point of maximum intensity to any other areas)?
- Is the patient otherwise ill or well?

Note: Much space is devoted in standard medical textbooks to detailed descriptions of the various heart murmurs and their pathological significance. However, this knowledge is of no use if you are unable to hear a murmur in the first place and describe it accurately. In any case, assessing the significance of a heart murmur usually requires specialist skill and experience. I therefore suggest that any patient with a previously undiagnosed heart murmur should be referred for specialist investigation (urgently if they are complaining of cardiac symptoms).

PROCEDURE:

Listen to these four areas again using the bell of your stethoscope. When you listen at the apex with the bell, lean the patient over to the left slightly as shown in Figure 12.

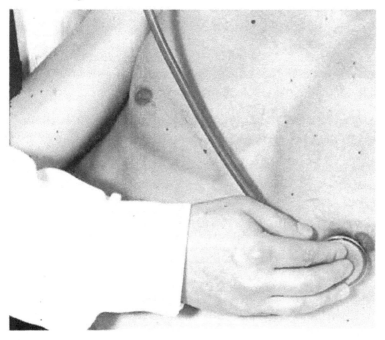

Figure 12

Sit the patient forward and listen at the left sternal edge with the diaphragm, with the patient holding their breath in expiration as shown in Figure 13.

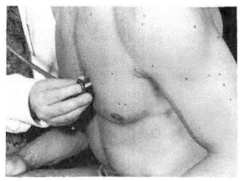

Figure 13

Hints and tips

Placing the patient in certain positions (leaning to the left, leaning forward) makes some murmurs easier to hear.

PROCEDURE:

Listen to the base of the lungs on the left and the right (Figure 14).

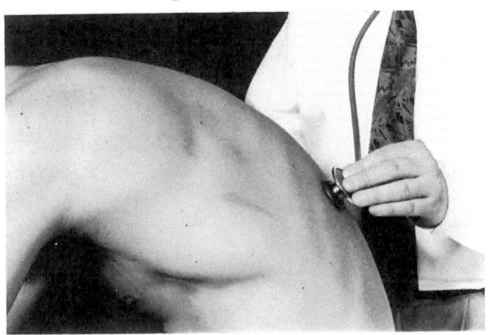

Figure 14

Hints and tips

Patients with pulmonary oedema (e.g. those with left heart failure or mitral stenosis) collect fluid in their lungs. When sitting upright, this fluid tends to collect at the lung bases and produces a crackling sound heard through the stethoscope when the patient breathes in.

Rub a few strands of your own hair between finger and thumb next to your ear. The crackles of pulmonary oedema sound just like this. If you think you do hear crackles at the lung bases, ask the patient to have a good cough then listen again. If the sounds disappear, pulmonary oedema was not the cause.

PROCEDURE:

Feel over the sacrum for pitting oedema (Figure 15)

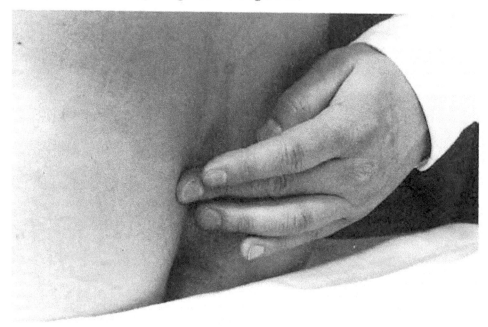

Figure 15

Hints and tips

Patients with gross peripheral oedema (such as those with severe right sided heart failure) accumulate fluid in the subcutaneous tissues around the sacrum if they sit for any length of time. You can assess this by pressing firmly on the skin over the sacrum for one minute and seeing if, when you take your finger away, there is a dent left behind that takes some time to go away. If there is, the patient is said to have 'pitting oedema'.

PROCEDURE:

Lie the patient back and try to find the dorsalis pedis (Figure 16a) and posterior tibial (Figure 16b) pulses in the feet

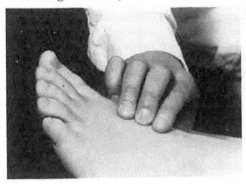 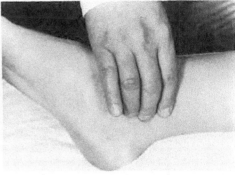

Figure 16a   Figure 16b

Hints and tips

Before you feel for the foot pulses, look at the colour of the feet and feel the toes to give you an impression of how good the peripheral circulation is (blue and cold suggests poor perfusion). Look also for signs of serious lack of blood supply such as small patches of blackness (gangrene) on the toes or under the foot.

As you feel the pulses, compare sides.

The dorsalis pedis pulse can usually be found just lateral to the tendons running to the big toe. The posterior tibial pulse can be found approximately midway between the tip of the medial malleolus and the heel.

A small proportion of people do not actually have a dorsalis pedis pulse (but, if healthy, should nevertheless have well perfused feet).

Two tips:

- Do not press too hard.
- Do not keep feeling for the pulse once you have found it; it will probably just seem to disappear again.

Note: If the foot pulses are present and equal and the feet are well perfused, there is not much point going on to assess the popliteal pulses (felt behind the knee in the middle of the crease with the knee slightly flexed) or the femoral pulses (palpated just below the middle of the inguinal ligament which runs from the anterior superior iliac spine to the pubic tubercle.)

PROCEDURE:

Feel the ankles for pitting oedema (Figure 17)

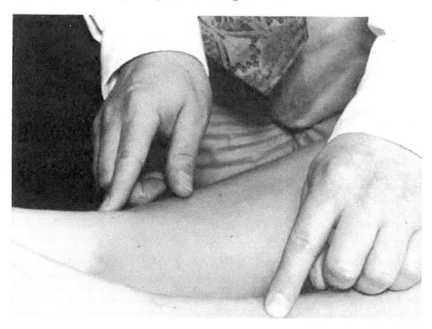

Figure 17

Hints and tips

As for sacral oedema, ankle oedema can be assessed by pressing with one finger on each leg over the tibia just above the malleoli for one minute and looking for 'pitting' when the fingers are removed.

If you do discover pitting oedema, repeat the test working up the leg until you find a level where there is no pitting. This gives an indication of the severity of the problem.

PROCEDURE:

Look at the fundi through an ophthalmoscope

Hints and tips

This procedure is fully described in Part 3.6, 'Using the ophthalmoscope and auriscope'.

Recording the Results of your Examination

Record your findings once the examination is completed

- General observations (well or unwell, breathless, colour, hands, etc)
- Pulse (rate, regularity, character)
- Peripheral pulses (normal or diminished)
- Blood pressure
- JVP (normal or raised)
- Peripheral oedema
- Apex beat (position, character)
- Thrills or heaves
- Heart sounds/added sounds/murmurs

In more or less standard medical shorthand, the entry in the notes for a person with a normal cardiovascular system might read:

Looks well

^{0} pallor

Hands NAD

Pulse 68/min reg

PPs present L=R

BP 120/70 JVP not raised

^{0} oedema

AB 5th ICS 10 cm from mid-line

HS 1 + 2 + nil

2.2 EXAMINING THE RESPIRATORY SYSTEM

Basic Routine

- Patient undressed to waist
- Observe general state
- Look at shape of chest
- Look at hands
- Face patient away from you and observe spine for obvious deformity
- Feel for swollen lymph glands in the neck and above the clavicles
- Assess chest expansion
- Assess tactile vocal fremitus in the upper, middle and lower chest posteriorly and under the arms, comparing sides
- Percuss the upper, middle and lower chest posteriorly and under the arms, comparing sides
- Listen to the upper, middle and lower chest posteriorly and under the arms with the bell of your stethoscope, comparing sides
- If there have been any abnormal findings, assess vocal resonance and whispering pectoriloquy
- Turn the patient to face you and assess the crico-sternal distance
- Feel the trachea in the suprasternal notch
- Feel the apex beat
- Assess chest expansion anteriorly
- Assess tactile vocal fremitus anteriorly, comparing sides
- Percuss the front of the chest, comparing sides
- Listen to the anterior chest with the bell of your stethoscope, comparing sides

STEP BY STEP

PROCEDURE:
Patient undressed to waist

Hints and tips
It may be necessary in some circumstances to examine the chest without removing clothes but, as in all clinical examination, proper exposure of the part

to be examined usually makes for a quicker, more efficient and thus, ultimately, less invasive interaction with the patient.

PROCEDURE:
Observe general state

Hints and tips
Do not stand too close.

Try to form a general impression (how ill, how anxious).

Observe the breathing (how fast, how laboured, any use of accessory muscles of respiration).

Look at the colour of the skin and mucous membranes (pale, cyanosed).

PROCEDURE:
Look at shape of chest

Hints and tips
Look for asymmetry, anatomical abnormality and hyperinflation.

PROCEDURE:
Look at hands

Hints and tips
Look for clubbing (see Part 2.1).

Look for peripheral cyanosis.

PROCEDURE:
Face patient away from you and observe spine for obvious deformity

Hints and tips
Look for asymmetries and abnormalities of contour that may affect the dimensions of the thoracic cavity.

PROCEDURE:
Feel for swollen lymph glands in the neck and above the clavicles

Hints and tips
This procedure is described in detail in Part 3.2.

PROCEDURE:

Assess chest expansion

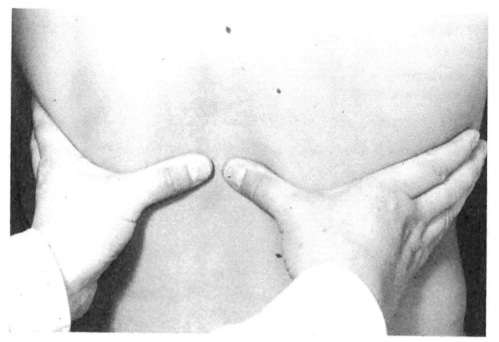

Figure 18a

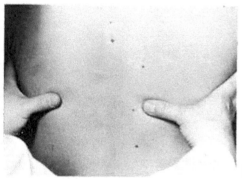

Figure 18b

Hints and tips

Ask the patient to take a deep breath and observe the expansion of the chest, looking for asymmetry. In most cases, the side that moves less is the side with the pathology.

Then, as the patient breathes out, place your hands at the bottom of their rib cage on each side and, with your fingers holding on firmly, bring your thumbs together in the mid-line (Figure 18a).

Ask the patient to take a good deep breath and allow your thumbs to be pulled apart from each other by the expansion of the chest (Figure 18b). Look for any asymmetry of movement. This method allows you to make a crude quantitative assessment of chest expansion and usually shows up any asymmetric movement. You can, of course, use a fabric tape measure to obtain a more accurate measurement of chest expansion.

PROCEDURE:
Assess tactile vocal fremitus in the upper, middle and lower chest posteriorly and under the arms comparing sides

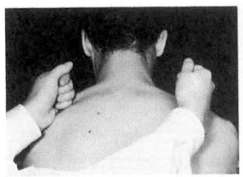

Figure 19a

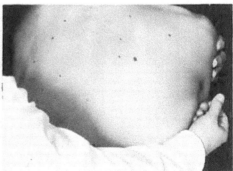

Figure 19b

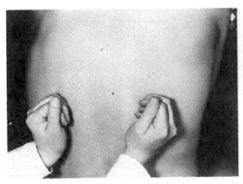

Figure 19c

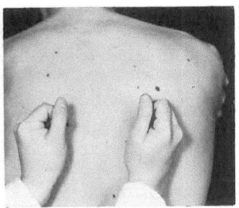

Figure 19d

Hints and tips

During this and the rest of the examination of the posterior chest, it is helpful to ask the patient to cross their arms in front of their chest and rest their hands on opposite shoulders. This gets the scapulae out of the way.

If you place your hand on someone's chest and ask them to speak, you will feel a vibration transmitted through the chest wall. This vibration has been labelled 'Tactile Vocal Fremitus' (TVF).

To assess TVF, place a sensitive part of your hands (e.g. the ulnar edge) on the patient's chest symmetrically either side of the spine near the top (Figure 19a) and ask them to say '99'. The vibration should feel more or less the same strength on both sides.

Repeat the test with your hands mid way down the chest (Figure 19b), at the bottom of the chest (Figure 19c) and under the arms (Figure 19d).

Differences in the strength of vibration felt can be caused by a variety of pathologies. These are summarized in the table at the end of Part 2.2.

PROCEDURE:

Percuss the upper, middle and lower chest and under the arms, comparing sides

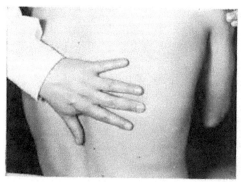
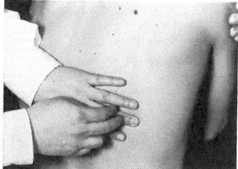

Figure 20a   Figure 20b

Hints and tips

It may take a lot of practice before you are satisfied with your percussion technique. The basic idea is simple: tap the chest with a finger and see if it sounds hollow or dull. For most people, it is easier to produce a clear sound by using the middle finger of one hand placed against the patient's skin as a sounding board (Figure 20a) and the middle finger of the other hand as a hammer (Figure 20b).

You will produce a clearer sound if i): the finger on the patient's skin is pressing down firmly, and ii): the movement of the striking finger is generated at the **elbow**, leaving the wrist floppy. In other words, the striking finger should fall on the pressing finger simply due to the action of gravity and not by the use of your wrist flexors.

Remember, it does not actually matter whether you can produce a loud sound or not; the important thing is to hear the difference between a dull and hollow sound. It is helpful to practise your percussion skills on any available surface at any available opportunity.

Try not to get into the habit of tapping furiously several times in each area of the chest; repeated tapping merely serves to dampen the sound of preceding taps and may make interpretation of your findings difficult.

Percuss the upper, middle and lower chest and under the arms in the same places that you assessed TVF, comparing sides and looking for asymmetry. The significance of dull and hollow sounds is indicated in the table at the end of Part 2.2.

PROCEDURE:
Listen to the upper, middle and lower chest and under the arms with the bell of your stethoscope, comparing sides (Figure 21)

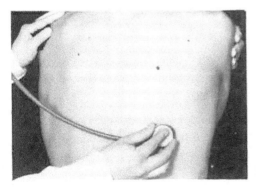

Figure 21

Hints and tips

You can use either side of the stethoscope to listen to breath sounds; most people find the bell slightly clearer.

Normal breath sounds are gentle and low-pitched with inspiration taking slightly longer than expiration and no perceptible break in the sounds between the in breath and the out breath. This normal pattern is called vesicular breathing.

You are listening for three things:

- The quality of the breath sounds
- Wheezes
- Crackles

Breath sounds

Mild inflammation of large airways can make the breath sounds rather coarse. Fibrosis (e.g. in fibrosing alveolitis) or consolidation (e.g. in pneumonia – you should refer to a standard textbook of medicine if you do not understand this term) will produce the phenomenon of 'bronchial breathing', heard over the affected area. Bronchial breathing is coarse and high-pitched with inspiration and expiration of equal length and a noticeable break in the sound between the in breath and the out breath. If you place your stethoscope over your own trachea in the suprasternal notch and listen, you will get a good idea of what 'bronchial breathing' sounds like.

Wheezes

Wheezes are produced by narrowing of the airways by muscle spasm (e.g. asthma), inflammation or obstruction.

Crackles

Crackles are caused by the production of too much mucus (e.g. chronic bronchitis) and by acute inflammation (e.g. acute bronchitis and pneumonia).

As for the heart, do not spend too long listening in any one area. Ask the patient to take moderately deep breaths through their open mouth. You can speed the process up by asking them to breathe in again before they have quite finished breathing out on the last breath.

PROCEDURE:

If there have been any abnormal findings, assess vocal resonance and whispering pectoriloquy

Hints and tips

Vocal resonance is the sound heard through a stethoscope applied to the chest when the patient *says* '99'. Whispering pectoriloquy is the sound heard through a stethoscope applied to the chest when a patient *whispers* '99'.

Pathologies that cause changes in TVF also cause parallel changes in vocal resonance and whispering pectoriloquy and therefore these two phenomena are usually only assessed if the rest of the examination has revealed an abnormality, particularly increased TVF in any area.

The technique is simple: place the stethoscope over the area of suspected abnormality and ask the patient to say '99'. Compare the sound produced with that over a 'normal' area. Repeat with the patient whispering '99'.

Changes in vocal resonance and whispering pectoriloquy mirror changes in TVF and have the same causes.

PROCEDURE:

Turn the patient to face you and assess the crico-sternal distance

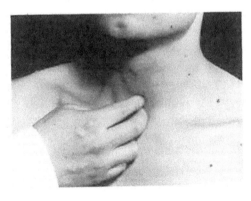

Figure 22

Hints and tips

In the average adult, it is usually possible to fit the tips of two fingers in the gap between the cricoid cartilage and the suprasternal notch (see Figure 22). In patients with chronic obstructive airways disease, the chest appears permanently overinflated and the crico-sternal gap diminishes.

PROCEDURE:

Feel the trachea in the suprasternal notch

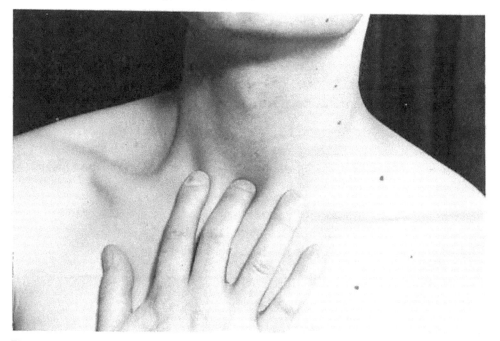

Figure 23

Hints and tips

If you press the tip of your middle finger into the suprasternal notch, you should just be able to feel the firm, rounded surface of the trachea right in the middle (see Figure 23). Do not press too hard since this can feel strange and uncomfortable for your patient. If serious lung pathology of one sort or another has pulled or pushed the trachea to one side, you will not feel the normal mid-line structure and your finger will seem to slip to one side.

Having said that, it is often quite difficult to feel the trachea in normal people and thus not too much weight should be placed on this sign by the inexperienced.

PROCEDURE:

Feel the apex beat

Hints and tips

This procedure has been described in detail in Part 2.1.

Gross lung pathology may cause a shift in the position of the whole mediastinum and thus alter the position of the apex beat. Remember, however, that an enlarged heart is a more likely cause of a displaced apex.

PROCEDURE:
Assess chest expansion anteriorly

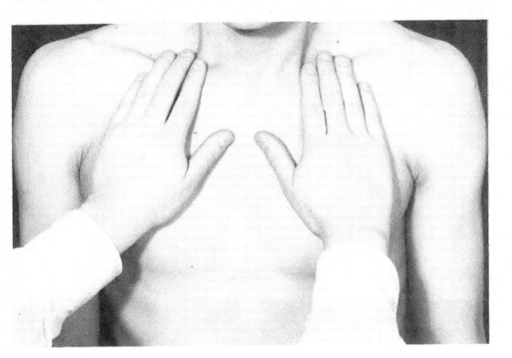

Figure 24

Hints and tips
As mentioned earlier, the side of the chest that moves less is the side containing the pathology. Asymmetric movement of the front of the chest can be easily assessed by placing your hands flat on the patient's chest, either side of the midline, and observing the relative movement of your thumbs as the patient breathes in (see Figure 24).

Remember that in examining the front of the chest you are (to all intents and purposes) examining the upper lobes of the lungs. Most of the back of the chest overlies the lower lobes.

PROCEDURE:

Assess tactile vocal fremitus (TVF) anteriorly, comparing sides

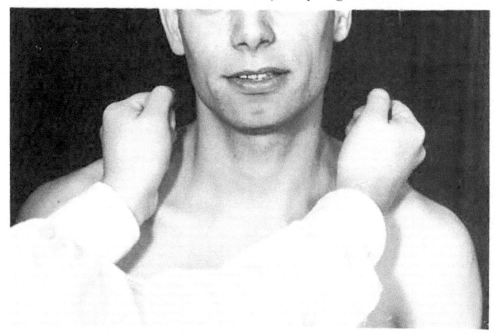

Figure 25a

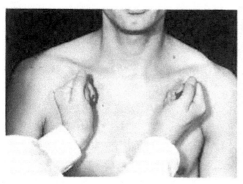

Figure 25b   Figure 25c

Hints and tips

The principles of this part of the examination have been described on pages 47–48. Assess TVF over the apices of the lungs (Figure 25a) and over a couple of other areas of the anterior chest (Figures 25b and c), comparing sides as usual.

PROCEDURE:

Percuss the front of the chest, comparing sides

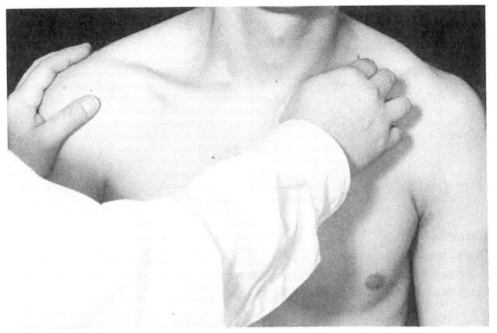

Figure 26a

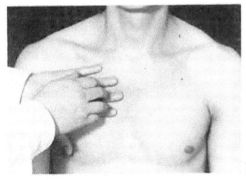

Figure 26b

Hints and tips

This procedure has already been described on page 48.

To percuss over the apex of each lung (Figure 26a), you can use the patient's clavicle as the 'sounding board', striking it directly with the 'hammer' finger. Percuss over the apices and over a couple of other areas of the anterior chest, comparing sides (Figure 26b).

PROCEDURE:

Listen to the anterior chest with the bell of your stethoscope, comparing sides (Figure 27)

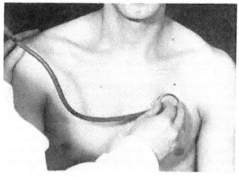

Figure 27

Hints and tips

The principles are the same as for listening to the back of the chest, described on pages 49–50. Listen over the apex of each lung in the supraclavicular fossae and over a couple of other areas of the anterior chest, comparing sides.

Note: As in all clinical examination, abnormal physical signs can only be interpreted in the light of the case history and the patient's general condition.

The following table lists some combinations of signs that may accompany certain significant lung pathologies:

TABLE 1

	Trachea	Expansion	TVF	PN	BS	Added Sounds
Consolidation or Fibrosis	Central	↓	↑	↓	Bronchial	Crackles
Pleural effusion	Pushed to opp. side	↓	↓	↓	↓	0
Lung collapse	Pulled to same side	↓	↓	↓	↓	0
Pneumothorax	Pushed to opp. side	↓	↓	↑	↓	0

Recording the Results of your Examination

Record your findings once the examination is completed

- General observations (well or unwell, breathless, cyanosed, clubbed fingers, swollen lymph nodes)
- Respiratory rate
- Trachea position
- Crico-sternal distance (C-S)
- Chest expansion (Exp)
- Tactile vocal fremitus (TVF)
- Percussion note (PN)
- Breath sounds (BS) (vesicular or bronchial)
- Added sounds (wheezes or crackles)

In more or less standard medical shorthand, the entry in the notes for a person with a normal respiratory system might read:

Looks well

^{0} SOB

^{0} cyanosis ^{0} clubbing ^{0} lymphad

Rate 15/min

Trachea central

C-S normal

Exp: NAD R=L

TVF: NAD R=L

PN: Resonant all areas

BS: Vesic + 0

2.3 EXAMINING THE GASTRO-INTESTINAL SYSTEM

Basic Routine

- Observe the general state of your patient
- Look at the hands
- Look at the eyes and mouth
- Help the patient to lie flat with arms at sides and abdomen fully exposed
- Look at the abdomen
- Palpate the abdomen superficially
- Palpate the abdomen more deeply
- Palpate for the liver
- Percuss to confirm liver size
- Palpate for the spleen
- Palpate for the kidneys
- Percuss the abdomen
- If indicated, check for shifting dullness
- Listen for bowel sounds with the diaphragm of the stethoscope
- Examine the hernial orifices
- If indicated, briefly examine external genitalia in males
- Consider the need for rectal examination

STEP BY STEP

PROCEDURE:
Observe the general state of your patient

Hints and tips
Do not stand too close.

Try to form a general impression (how ill, how thin, alert or confused).

Look at the colour of the skin and mucous membranes (jaundice, pallor).

Look for any unusual marks on the skin (e.g. spider naevi or Campbell de Morgan spots).

Note: Naevus means mark. A spider naevus is a visible arteriole with some capillaries spreading out from it like the legs of a spider. Its chief characteristic is that when you press on the centre, e.g. with the end of a capped biro, the blood (and thus the red colour) drains away. When you release the pressure, blood fills the 'legs' of the 'spider' from the centre outwards. Spider naevi are small and sometimes insignificant looking. Their cause is unknown and perfectly healthy people may have a few (up to six). They also sometimes appear in pregnancy. More than six 'spiders' in a person with risk factors for liver disease may suggest chronic liver damage.

Campbell de Morgan spots are bright red, slightly raised spots that appear on the chest, back and abdomen of people of advancing age. They have no sinister significance.

PROCEDURE:
Look at the hands

Hints and tips
Clubbing (see Part 2.1), very white nails and palmar erythema (a redness of the outer borders of the palms) are all associated with chronic liver disease.

Nails in bad condition and (particularly) nails whose convex surface is hollowed into a spoon shape (koilonychia) are associated with anaemia.

Note: Thickening of the palmar fascia with tethering of the skin of the palm to the flexor tendon of the fourth finger is known as **Dupuytren's contracture**. It is associated with cirrhosis of the liver but also occurs in normal people. It can be diagnosed by running your thumb across the upper palm, feeling for thickening of the subcutaneous tissue. In extreme cases the fourth and fifth fingers are pulled downward into permanent flexion.

PROCEDURE:
Look at the eyes and mouth

Hints and tips:
Look at the sclerae for the yellow tinge of jaundice and the conjunctivae for the pallor of anaemia.

Look at the mouth for the sore, cracked corners ('angular stomatitis') and smooth, sore red tongue that may accompany anaemia and some vitamin deficiencies.

Make a brief assessment of the state of the teeth and look at the tongue and inside of the cheeks for any growths or discoloured patches (e.g. firm white patches of precancerous 'leucoplakia' or the fragile, cottage cheesy, white lesions of candida).

PROCEDURE:
Help the patient to lie flat with arms at sides and abdomen fully exposed

Hints and tips
Be aware that many patients feel vulnerable lying flat on their back, especially with their abdomen bare! Do all you can to ensure the patient feels comfortable and safe (warm room, warm feet, a pillow under the knees to help keep the abdomen relaxed, etc).

PROCEDURE:
Look at the abdomen

Hints and tips:
Inspect the exposed abdomen carefully.

Old operation *scars* may give information not revealed in the history.

According to a traditional medical saying, a swollen abdomen may be caused by fat, flatus, faeces, fluid and (in women) by fibroids and a foetus. Abdominal tumours may also cause swelling.

People with chronic liver disease may have *sparse body hair*.

People with Cushing's syndrome may have discoloured purple *stretch marks* on their abdomen.

You might also notice:

Hernias; visible peristaltic movements; abnormal pulsations and dilated veins.

PROCEDURE:

Palpate the abdomen superficially (Figure 28)

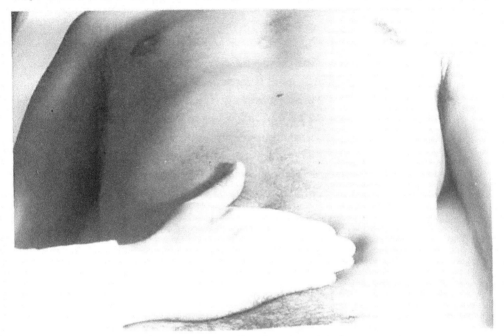

Figure 28

Hints and tips

Before laying a hand on the patient, you need to consider a number of points.

1   It can be quite disturbing, from the patient's point of view, to have someone looming over you and prodding your abdomen. Many practitioners thus find it helpful to kneel down beside the examination couch which places their head on the same level as the patient's and allows for a more relaxed use of the examining hand.

2   You should always check that your patient does not need to empty their bowels or bladder before you press on their abdomen – you otherwise risk discovering the answer the hard way.

3   You should always ask whether any particular areas of the abdomen are tender or painful and then do your best to start your palpation as far away from such areas as possible.

4   You should try to examine with warm hands. Confidence in your basic clinical skills helps keep your hands warm.

5 Keep your eyes on the patient's face while palpating to ensure that you do not miss any signs of discomfort.

6 Most practitioners consider that placing one hand flat on the abdomen and then pressing downwards by flexing the fingers at the metacarpophalangeal joints is the best way of palpating. Develop the habit of *concentrating* on the tactile information coming from your hands. Decide which part of each hand is most sensitive and focus your attention on this area whilst examining. The attitude is somewhat the same as when listening with rapt attention to a beautiful piece of music, except that in this case you are 'listening' to your hand.

7 It pays to palpate the abdomen in a systematic manner to make sure that you cover all areas (see Diagram 1 below). Feeling over each area in a diminishing clockwise spiral is a favoured approach.

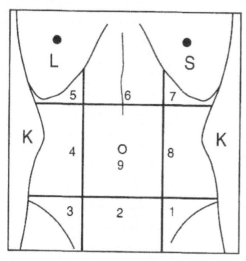

Diagram 1

1 Left Iliac fossa
2 Hypogastrium
3 Right Iliac fossa
4 Right lumbar
5 Right hypochondrium (hypo=below, chondrium=ribs)
6 Epigastrium
7 Left hypochondrium
8 Left lumbar
9 Umbilical

As you feel in each area, look for:

- **lumps;**
- **tenderness;**
- **guarding** (muscles going tight under the hand to protect from pain);
- **rigidity** (tense, hard, fixed contraction of abdominal muscles over an area of peritonitis. Patients with peritonitis will be obviously very ill).

PROCEDURE:
Palpate the abdomen more deeply (Figure 29)

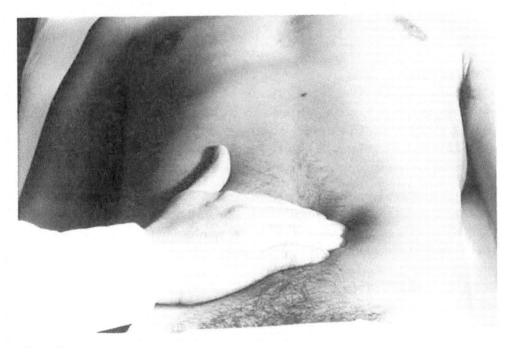

Figure 29

Hints and tips
Follow the same procedure as for superficial palpation, looking for the same things.

Make sure that you apply deep pressure in a progressive manner, not with a sudden push. The correct pressure for deep palpation is enough to cause mild discomfort in a healthy person.

PROCEDURE:

Palpate for the liver

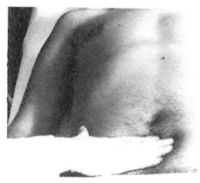 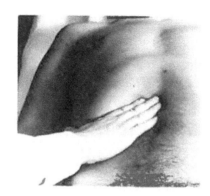

Figure 30a   Figure 30b

Hints and tips

In a healthy person, the liver is not palpable. However, in some conditions that cause liver enlargement, the increase in size is enormous. When feeling for an enlarged liver, therefore, palpation starts in the right iliac fossa (RIF) with the edge of the hand roughly parallel to the right rib margin. Feeling for an enlarged liver (or spleen or kidney) requires moderately deep palpation.

Watch the patient's breathing as you feel. The liver edge will move downwards during inspiration and, if the liver is enlarged, you will feel its edge push against your hand as the patient breathes in. If you feel nothing in the RIF, move your hand *up* towards the costal margin a few centimetres as the patient breathes *out* and be pressing *in* again in time for the next *in* breath (Figure 30a). Repeat the same procedure three or four more times until your hand is pressing in just below the costal margin (Figure 30b).

If you think you have felt an enlarged liver, try to decide whether it is hard or firm, smooth or irregular in surface contour, pulsatile or non pulsatile and tender or not tender.

Primary and secondary cancers (including blood cancers), cirrhosis, infections of various types and heart failure may all cause liver enlargement.

PROCEDURE:
Percuss to confirm liver size

Hints and tips
The liver is a large organ and its normal surface markings are a triangle bounded by the nipples, the anterior costal margin and a line dropped perpendicular from the right nipple to the costal margin (Figure 31).

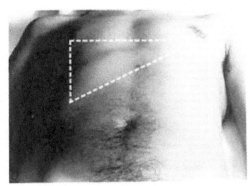

Figure 31

It can thus be helpful to percuss (see Part 2.2) from the nipple line and downwards over the costal margin on to the abdomen to help confirm your palpatory findings. In a normal person, the slightly dull percussion note over the liver changes to a more hollow sound over the abdomen, just below the costal margin. See Figure 32.

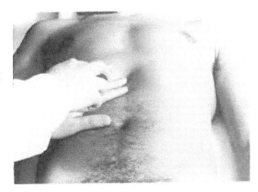

Figure 32

PROCEDURE:
Palpate for the spleen

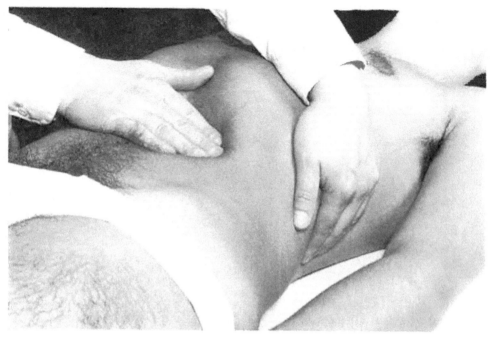

Figure 33

Hints and tips

Like the liver, a normal spleen is impalpable but disease can cause massive enlargement. However, a diseased spleen enlarges diagonally in the general direction of the RIF rather than straight down and so, once again, the examining hand starts in the RIF but with the fingers angled towards the left costal margin. You examine progressively upwards towards the left costal margin, palpating in inspiration and moving your hand during expiration since the spleen, like the liver, moves downwards during inspiration.

It may help to put your free hand behind the patient's lower rib cage on the left (see Figure 33), gently inclining them towards you, as you feel for the spleen with the other hand. It should be possible to feel a notch on the surface of an enlarged spleen and this, plus the fact that you can not get your fingers above it, can help to distinguish an enlarged spleen from other abdominal swellings. Large spleens usually suggest blood cancers or infections (including malaria and glandular fever).

PROCEDURE:

Palpate for the kidneys

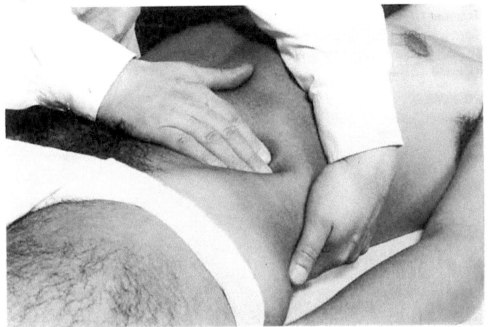

Figure 34

Hints and tips

As you can see from Figure 34, you use both hands to feel for an enlarged kidney. The left hand is placed in the patient's renal angle (i.e. the gap between the rib cage and the pelvis) and the right hand is placed anteriorly, pushing inwards. As the patient takes a deep breath, the posterior (left) hand pushes upwards quite sharply. If the kidney is enlarged, it will then be felt pushing against the anterior (right) hand. It is sometimes possible to feel the lower pole of a normal kidney using this technique in a thin person. Pathological enlargement may be caused by a number of conditions including renal tumours and polycystic kidney disease.

PROCEDURE:
Percuss the abdomen

Hints and tips
There is no need to percuss the abdomen routinely. If the abdomen is swollen or if you palpate a mass, percussion is used to provide more information on size, shape and density.

PROCEDURE:
If indicated, check for shifting dullness

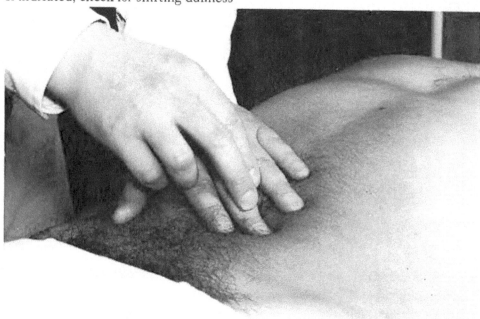

Figure 35a

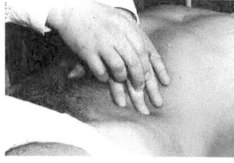

Figure 35b

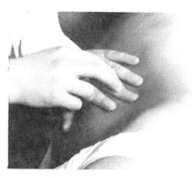

Figure 35c

Hints and tips

Patients with raised pressure in their portal venous system (e.g. patients with serious chronic liver disease) may develop ascites (oedema in the abdomen). Since ascites fluid is freely mobile within the abdominal cavity, it is possible to elicit the sign of shifting dullness in people with abdomens distended by ascites.

The underlying principle of the test is simple. When a person with ascites lies flat on their back, the ascites fluid collects equally in both flanks. When they roll on to one side, all the fluid collects on that side.

Thus, with the patient lying on their back, you percuss the abdomen, starting in the middle and working away from you until you reach the point (over the fluid) where the percussion note becomes dull (Figures 35a and 35b). Keeping your finger on this point, ask the patient to roll over towards you, wait a few seconds and percuss again over the same spot (Figure 35c). If the patient has ascites, the fluid will all have run towards the side s/he has rolled towards and so the percussion note under your finger will change from dull to hollow. This effect is known as shifting dullness (a name used by some medical students for their teachers, and by some medical teachers for their students).

PROCEDURE:

Listen for bowel sounds with the diaphragm of the stethoscope (Figure 36)

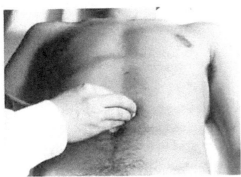
Figure 36

Hints and tips

Once again, auscultation of the abdomen is really only of use in patients with distinct abdominal symptoms. You need only listen in one place and you are listening for just two things:

i) Are there any bowel sounds at all? (It may take 20 seconds or so to hear bowel sounds in a normal patient. In patients with generalized peritonitis, bowel sounds stop altogether.)

ii) Do the bowel sounds sound normal? (In patients with bowel obstruction, bowel sounds become much more active and take on a harsh, metallic quality usually referred to as 'tinkling'.)

Note that in patients with occlusive vascular disease, it is sometimes possible to hear whooshing noises ('bruits') over the femoral and renal arteries.

PROCEDURE:
Examine the hernial orifices

Hints and tips
This procedure is described in detail in Part 3.3.

PROCEDURE:
If indicated, briefly examine the external genitalia in males

Hints and tips
In cases of suspected indirect inguinal hernia in males (see Part 3.3), it is obviously necessary to examine the scrotum. Any complaint of testicular or scrotal swelling also demands brief observation and palpation of the scrotum and testes. Your decision to perform such examination must be guided by the policies in force in your training clinic and by the advice of senior clinic tutors.

PROCEDURE:
Consider the need for rectal examination

Hints and tips
It could be argued that *anyone* with a case history meriting full abdominal examination should have a rectal examination. It is certainly *absolutely necessary* for anyone complaining of rectal bleeding, a change of bowel habit or (males) problems urinating to have a rectal examination by an experienced clinician.

The practical skill of rectal examination must be learned in an appropriate clinical setting and thus will not be described here. For some practitioners, however, the invasive nature of the procedure and the limited opportunity to develop the necessary skills during training together form a case for referral of all patients requiring rectal examination to a doctor with appropriate experience.

Recording the Results of your Examination

Record your findings once the examination is completed.

- General observations
- Hands
- Mouth
- Signs of chronic liver disease
- Is abdomen soft
- Any tenderness or guarding
- Any rigidity
- Any palpable masses
- Any organ enlargement (LKKS)
- Bowel sounds (BS)
- Hernial orifices (HO)
- External genitalia
- Rectal examination (PR)

In more or less standard medical shorthand, the entry in the notes for a person with a normal gastro-intestinal system might read:

Looks well

^{0} pallor ^{0} jaundice

Mouth NAD

Abdo soft

^{0} tenderness ^{0} guarding

^{0}L ^{0}K ^{0}K ^{0}S

^{0} masses

BS normal

HOs normal

Ext. gen NAD

PR NAD

2.4 EXAMINING THE NERVOUS SYSTEM

Basic Routine

- Assess consciousness, orientation and memory
- Look for tremors and gross weakness of upper limbs
- Test co-ordination
- Assess function of cranial nerves II–XII:
    Visual acuity (II)
    Peripheral visual fields (II)
    Pupils: symmetry, size and reactions to light and accommodation (II, III)
    Eye movements (III, IV, VI)
    Nystagmus (cerebellar or vestibular)
    Fundi (II)
    Trigeminal (V) sensation (including corneal reflex)
    Trigeminal (V) motor function (e.g. opening mouth)
    Facial nerve (VII) function (muscles of facial expression)
    Hearing (VIII), including Weber and Rinne tests
    Ask patient to say *aaaaah* – look for symmetrical movement of uvula (IX)
    Coughing and swallowing and gag reflex (IX, X)
    Ask patient to stick out their tongue (XII)
    Test strength of sternomastoid and trapezius (XI)
- Observe upper limbs for muscle wasting or fasciculation
- Assess upper limb tone
- Assess upper limb power
- Observe lower limbs for muscle wasting or fasciculation
- Assess lower limb tone
- Assess lower limb power
- Elicit tendon jerks and plantar responses
- Test vibration sense in feet
- Test position sense in feet
- Briefly test sensitivity to light touch and pinprick
- Perform Romberg test
- Watch patient walk

STEP BY STEP

PROCEDURE:
Assess consciousness, orientation and memory

Hints and tips
Is the person conscious? Do they know who they are and where they are; do they know what year and day of the week it is? The assessment of cognitive function is described in more detail in Part 2.6.

PROCEDURE:
Look for tremors and gross weakness of upper limbs

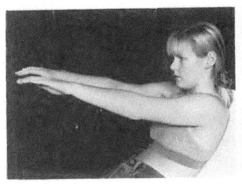 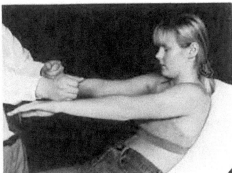

Figure 37a   Figure 37b

Hints and tips
Ask the patient to hold their arms steadily out in front of them (Figure 37a); look for tremors and for drift of one arm downwards or upwards. After about 30 seconds, ask them to close their eyes while you give a brief push downwards on their wrists (Figure 37b). They should resist the downward pressure quite easily and their arms should quickly return to more or less the original position.

Then ask the patient to open their eyes and, still keeping their arms out in front, to make piano playing movements with their fingers. This is hard to do if you have any gross weakness or co-ordination problem.

PROCEDURE:
Test co-ordination

Hints and tips
Ask the patient to touch their nose with their right forefinger and then to touch

your forefinger, which you hold in the air about half a metre in front of them. Ask them to repeat this movement, back and forth, as quickly and accurately as possible whilst you move your finger around (so that they have to 'change direction' from time to time). Repeat with the patient using their left forefinger (Figure 38a).

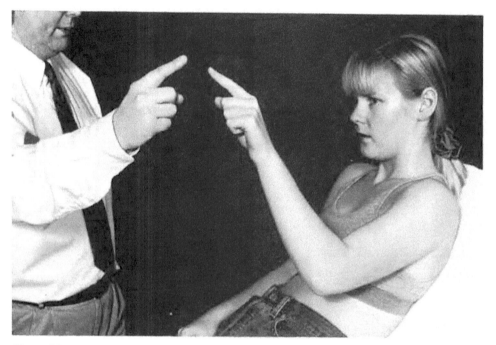

Figure 38a

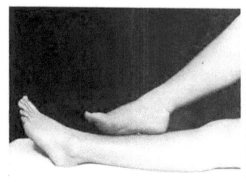

Figure 38b

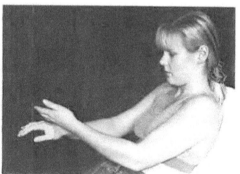

Figure 38c

Ask the patient to draw the heel of one leg slowly and accurately up the shin of their opposite leg, from ankle to knee and then back down again. Repeat the test for the other leg (Figure 38b).

Ask the patient to show you rapid alternating movements with each hand, such as imitating the action of using a screwdriver or tapping the back of one hand with the palm, and then the back of the other, alternating as quickly as possible (Figure 38c).

Obvious inability to perform these tests (taking account of age, poor sight, restricted movement due to arthritis, etc) would suggest cerebellar dysfunction. Patients with cerebellar disease develop gross tremor (intention tremor) when trying to perform complex tasks such as the 'finger/nose' and 'heel/shin' tests. They are also unable to perform rapid alternating movements. The inability to perform rapid alternating movements is referred to as dysdiadochokinesia.

PROCEDURE:
Assess function of cranial nerves II–XII:

Hints and tips
Learning to test the cranial nerves always seems a daunting task but, if you think about it, it is usually obvious whether the cranial nerves are working properly. All you have to do is observe closely when you first meet your client. Can they see where they are going? Do they complain of tunnel vision? Do both eyes move together and have they got a squint? Do their pupils look symmetrical and do they seem to react to light and accommodation? Do their eyes flicker rapidly back and forth as they look at you? Do they open and close their mouth normally? Do they have a full and more or less symmetrical range of facial expressions? Can they hear what you are saying to them? Do they seem to be coughing and swallowing normally (watch as they clear their throat before speaking)? Is their tongue allowing them to speak normally? Are they able to shrug their shoulders?

In practice, few practitioners (except neurologists) bother to test the cranial nerves in great detail once they see that there is no gross abnormality; so it would be a shame if basic examination of the cranial nerves were to become a 'no-go' area for you.

Here, once again, is a brief summary of the basic routine:

- Visual acuity (II)
- Peripheral visual fields (II)
- Pupils: symmetry, size and reactions to light and accommodation (II, III)
- Eye movements (III, IV, VI)
- Nystagmus (cerebellar or vestibular)
- Fundi (II)
- Trigeminal (V) sensation (including corneal reflex)
- Trigeminal (V) motor function (e.g. opening mouth)
- Facial nerve (VII) function (muscles of facial expression)
- Hearing (VIII), including Weber and Rinne tests
- Ask patient to say *aaaaah* – look for symmetrical movement of uvula (IX)
- Coughing and swallowing and gag reflex (IX, X)
- Ask patient to stick out tongue (XII)
- Test strength of sternomastoid and trapezius (XI)

We will now consider each of these tests in turn.

PROCEDURE:
Test visual acuity (II)

Hints and tips
Test the ability to read print at a distance (any convenient large print will do) and close up (a book or magazine). If your client wears glasses or contact lenses, they should keep these on. If you consider your vision to be normal and the patient appears to see as well as you on these tests, then you can reasonably assume that the patient is not suffering a major defect of visual acuity. However, you should be aware that visual acuity can only be tested accurately using standardized test charts (e.g. Snellen's).

All patients with decreased visual acuity should be referred for expert assessment.

PROCEDURE:
Test peripheral visual fields (II)

Hints and tips
Standing or sitting about a metre away from your patient with your head on the same level as theirs, ask them to look you straight in the eyes. Hold your arms

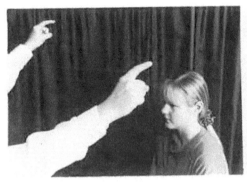

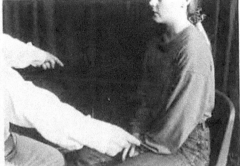

Figure 39a   Figure 39b

out to the side with your fingers half way between you and your client and, with your arms first as high up as they can go (Figure 39a) and then as low down as they can go (Figure 39b), check that your patient can see your fingers wiggling at the edges of their visual field as clearly as you can, both on the left and the right.

Patients with obvious or gross visual field defects should be referred for expert assessment.

PROCEDURE:
Test pupils: symmetry, size and reactions to light and accommodation (II, III)

Hints and tips:
Observe the size, shape and symmetry of the pupils.

Note whether either eyelid is drooping (III).

Shine a narrow torch beam twice into each pupil. The first time, check that the pupil being shone into contracts; the second time, watch the other pupil and check that it contracts 'consensually' (at the same time).

Ask the patient to fix their gaze on some distant object and then ask them to change their focus to a finger held up directly in front of them, about half a metre away. The eyeballs should turn inwards and the pupils constrict as they 'accommodate' to the closer object.

PROCEDURE:
Test eye movements (III, IV, VI) (Figure 40)

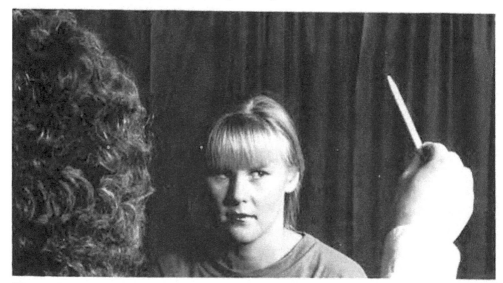

Figure 40

Hints and tips
Stand or sit directly opposite your client about one metre away and ask them to follow with their eyes the tip of a pen as you draw a circle in the air about 75cm in diameter and half a metre away from them. Look to see if their eyes move symmetrically in every direction of gaze. If a squint appears in any direction, ask the patient if they see double.

PROCEDURE:
Check for nystagmus (cerebellar or vestibular)

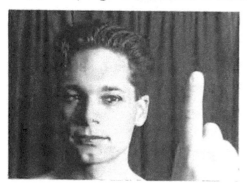

Figure 41

Hints and tips

Though this is not exactly a test of cranial nerve function, it is convenient to perform it at this point in your assessment.

Hold your finger about a metre away from your client directly in line with their nose and then move it to the side so that the eyeballs swivel about 30 degrees away from the midline (Figure 41). Ask them to hold their gaze like this for about a minute. Look carefully to see if the eyes start jerking sideways. Repeat with the gaze in the opposite direction.

Cerebellar lesions cause fast jerking movements towards the direction of gaze. The jerks are apparent when looking in either direction but they are more pronounced when the patient looks towards the side of the cerebellar pathology.

Vestibular lesions cause fast jerking movements in one direction only – away from the side of the lesion.

PROCEDURE:
Examine fundi (II)

Hints and tips
This procedure is described in detail in Part 3.6, 'Using the ophthalmoscope and auriscope'.

PROCEDURE:
Test Trigeminal (V) sensation (including corneal reflex)

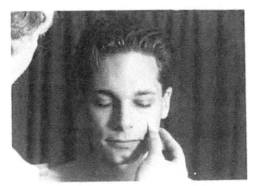

Figure 42

Hints and tips

Ask the patient to close their eyes and then use a small piece of cotton wool to brush lightly against the skin of the face on the left and right forehead, left and right cheek and left and right chin. Ask the patient to say 'yes' each time they feel a light touch (Figure 42).

Then elicit the corneal reflex. This is done by twisting a little bit of cotton wool into a fine wisp and touching the edge of each cornea (overlying the coloured part of the eye) lightly, approaching from the side. The patient will blink sharply if the reflex is intact.

It is important to approach the cornea from the side since a head on approach will probably cause the patient to blink before the cornea itself is touched.

PROCEDURE:

Test Trigeminal (V) motor function (e.g. opening mouth)

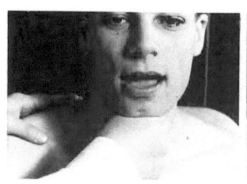 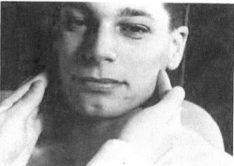

Figure 43a   Figure 43b

Hints and tips

Ask your client to open their jaw against the resistance of your hand placed under their chin (Figure 43a). Then ask them to clench their teeth hard whilst you feel the bulk of the masseter muscle on each side (Figure 43b).

The jaw should open symmetrically and the masseters should be of equal bulk.

PROCEDURE:

Test facial nerve (VII) function (muscles of facial expression) (Figure 44)

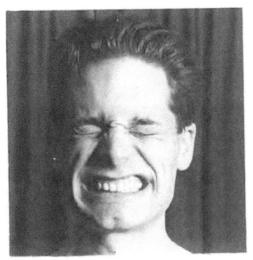

Figure 44

Hints and tips

Ask your client to raise their eyebrows, screw their eyes up tight, show their teeth and puff out their cheeks (preferably not at the same time).

All these facial movements should be more or less strong and symmetrical.

PROCEDURE:

Test hearing (VIII), including Weber and Rinne tests

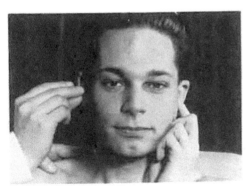

Figure 45

Hints and tips:

Ask the patient to block one ear with a finger. Test the hearing in the other by gently rubbing your fingers together a few centimetres away from the open ear. Repeat on the other side. See Figure 45.

If you suspect a hearing loss, perform Rinne's test and Weber's test with a tuning fork as follows:

Rinne's Test

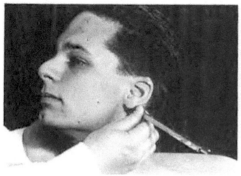
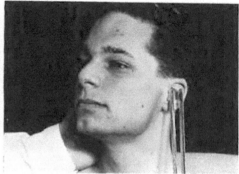

Figure 46a   Figure 46b

Set a 'medical' tuning fork vibrating by hitting it gently against your knee. Place the base on the mastoid process of the 'good' side (Figure 46a). Ask the patient to tell you when the sound stops. As soon as they tell you, hold the vibrating end of the fork next to the ear-hole and ask if they can hear the sound (Figure 46b). Repeat on the other side.

Weber's Test (Figure 47)

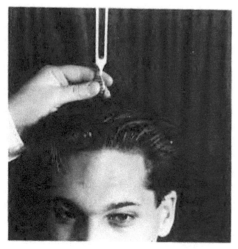

Figure 47

Set the tuning fork vibrating quite strongly and place it in the middle of the top of the patient's head. Ask whether the sound seems equally loud in both ears or is louder in one than the other.

Note: These tests often cause confusion but they are useful in confirming a suspicion of conductive deafness, for example in otitis media. (Assessment of nerve deafness usually requires specialist referral.)

Normal people hear sound better when it is conducted via the air into the ear and on to the tympanic membrane. Patients with conductive deafness tend to hear sound better when it is transmitted directly through bone. In other words, for normal people, air conduction is better than bone conduction. In patients suffering from conductive deafness, bone conduction is better than air conduction.

Thus, in Rinne's test, a normal person will still hear the tuning fork held by the ear hole even after they have ceased to hear the sound of the fork pressed on to the mastoid process. However, a patient with conductive deafness will not hear the tuning fork held by the ear-hole once they have ceased to hear the sound of the fork pressed on to the mastoid on the affected side.

In Weber's test, a normal person will hear the sound of the tuning fork equally in both ears. A patient with conductive deafness will hear the sound more distinctly *on the affected side.*

If there is any doubt about the cause, all patients with hearing loss should be referred for expert assessment.

PROCEDURE:
Ask patient to say *aaaaah* – look for symmetrical movement of uvula (IX)

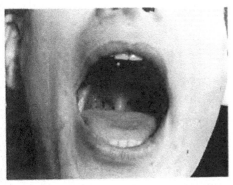

Figure 48

Hints and tips

Ask the patient to open their mouth wide. Shine a torch in and ask them to say *aaaaah* (Figure 48). Look for symmetry in the movement of the uvula.

PROCEDURE:

Test coughing and swallowing and gag reflex (IX, X)

Hints and tips

Make sure that your patient can cough and swallow normally.

Test the gag reflex by gently touching the back of the pharynx with a tongue depressor.

PROCEDURE:

Ask patient to stick out their tongue (XII)

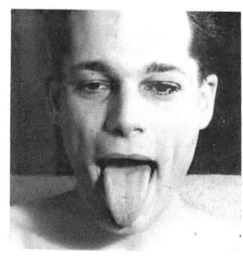

Figure 49

Hints and tips

The tongue should not deviate to one side or the other (Figure 49). If it does, the deviation will be towards the side of any XIIth nerve lesion. Look also for any unusual writhing movements or wasting of the tongue.

PROCEDURE:

Test strength of sternomastoid and trapezius (XI)

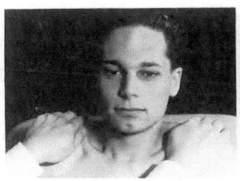

Figure 50a

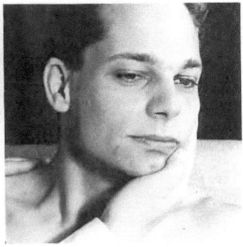

Figure 50b

Hints and tips

Ask your client to shrug their shoulders upwards against a downward pressure from your hands placed on top of their shoulders (over trapezius). Both sides should be equally strong (Figure 50a).

Test the XIth nerve further by asking your client to turn their head (as if to place their chin on their shoulder) to each side against resistance from your hand (Figure 50b).

PROCEDURE:

Observe upper limbs for muscle wasting or fasciculation

Hints and tips

Look carefully for asymmetry of muscle bulk in the upper limbs.

Look also for small rippling movements of muscles (called fasciculation) which may occur when anterior horn cells are destroyed (e.g. motor neurone disease).

PROCEDURE:

Assess upper limb tone

Hints and tips

Assess upper limb tone by moving each of the patient's arms around so that you flex and extend the wrist and the elbow (Figure 51). It is important that the patient relaxes as much as possible. It is usually more helpful to say 'give me your arm' than 'relax your arm' when testing upper limb tone.

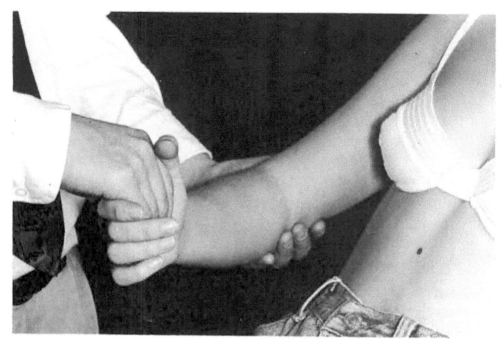

Figure 51

A marked increase in tone would suggest an upper motor neurone (UMN) (pyramidal tract) lesion of the opposite side (e.g. stroke) or an extrapyramidal problem (e.g. Parkinsonism).

Increased tone caused by UMN lesions may be accompanied by a 'clasp knife' response, i.e. a sudden decrease in muscle tone when the affected limb is flexed beyond a certain point.

Patients with Parkinson's disease have a rapid tremor superimposed on their increased muscle tone which gives rise to a jerky 'cogwheeling' effect. This is most clearly felt by holding the patient's hand and alternately pronating and supinating the forearm.

Marked hypotonia (decreased muscle tone) suggests a lower motor neurone lesion (or possibly cerebellar disease). Patients who have recently had a stroke may also have decreased muscle tone on the affected side for a time.

PROCEDURE:
Assess upper limb power

Hints and tips
Assess upper limb power by asking for and resisting the following movements, looking for differences in power between sides.

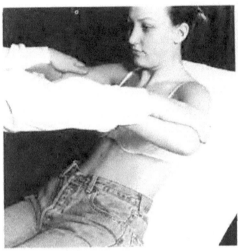

Figure 52a. 'Raise your arms out to the sides with your elbows bent.'

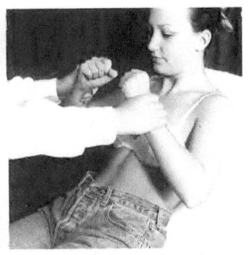

Figure 52b. 'Pull me towards you.'

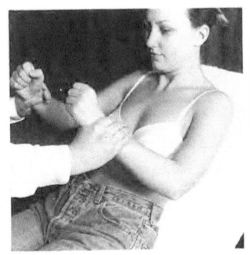

Figure 52c. 'Push me away.'

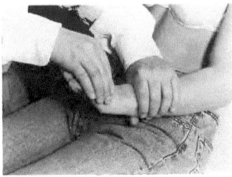

Figure 52d. 'Cock your wrists up.'

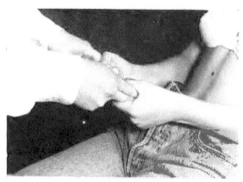 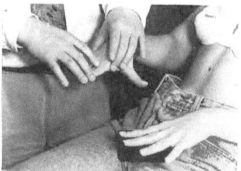

Figure 52e. 'Grip two of my fingers tightly and do not let me pull them away.'

Figure 52f. 'Spread your fingers apart – do not let me squeeze them together.'

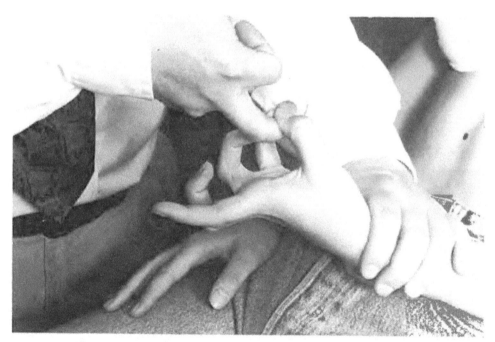

Figure 52g. 'Squeeze your little finger and thumb together – do not let me pull them apart.'

The section on *myotomes* at the end of Part 2.4 contains information to help you interpret the results of these tests.

PROCEDURE:

Observe lower limbs for muscle wasting or fasciculation

Hints and tips

Look carefully for asymmetry of muscle bulk in the lower limbs.

Look also for irregular small movements of muscles (called fasciculation) which may occur when anterior horn cells are damaged (e.g. in motor neurone disease).

PROCEDURE:

Assess lower limb tone

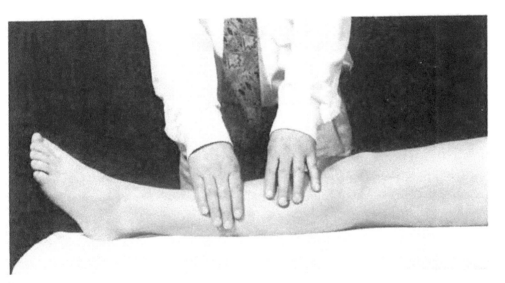

Figure 53

Hints and tips

Assess lower limb tone by rolling each leg gently from side to side with the patient lying down and relaxed (Figure 53).

Alternatively, ask the patient to relax and then, with your hands underneath a leg just above the knee, give a quick flick upwards and watch the heel (Figure 54).

In a relaxed leg with normal tone, the heel will stay in contact with the bed. In a limb with increased tone, the heel will lift off the bed.

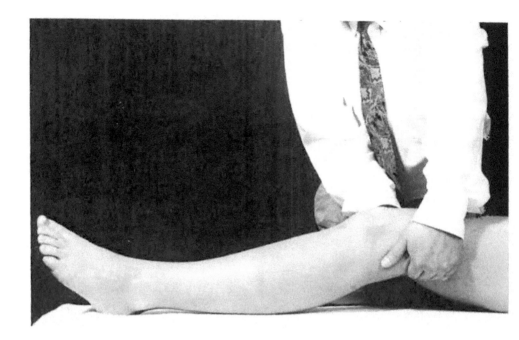

Figure 54

A marked increase in tone would suggest an upper motor neurone (UMN) (pyramidal tract) lesion of the opposite side (e.g. stroke) or an extrapyramidal problem (e.g. Parkinsonism).

Increased tone caused by UMN lesions may be accompanied by a 'clasp knife' response, i.e. a sudden decrease in muscle tone when the affected limb is flexed beyond a certain point. Patients with Parkinson's disease have a rapid tremor superimposed on their increased muscle tone which gives rise to a jerky 'cogwheeling' effect.

Marked hypotonia (decreased muscle tone) suggests a lower motor neurone (LMN) lesion (or possibly cerebellar disease). Patients who have recently had a stroke may also have decreased muscle tone on the affected side for a time.

PROCEDURE:
Assess lower limb power

Hints and tips
Assess lower limb power using the following resisted movements, comparing sides as you go:

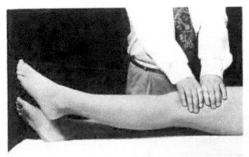

Figure 55a. 'Lift your leg off the bed and keep it there as I push down.'

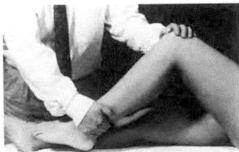

Figure 55b. 'Pull your heel up towards your bottom.'

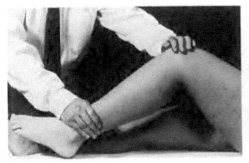

Figure 55c. 'Straighten your leg out.'

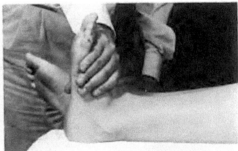

Figure 55d. 'Cock your ankle upwards against my hand.'

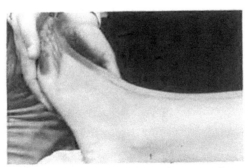

Figure 55e. 'Push your foot downwards against my hand.'

The section on *myotomes* at the end of Part 2.4 contains information to help you interpret the results of these tests.

PROCEDURE:
Elicit tendon jerks and plantar responses

Hints and tips
Test the reflexes in the following order:

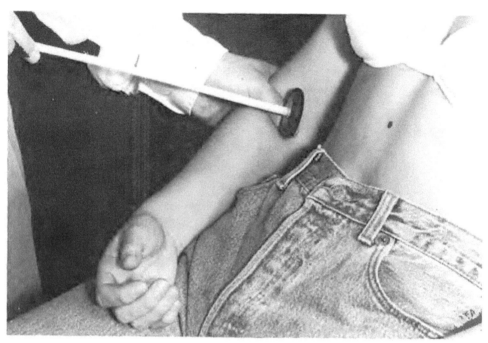

Figure 56a. Elicit biceps jerk on both sides

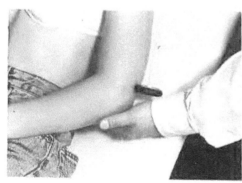

Figure 56b. Elicit triceps jerk on both sides

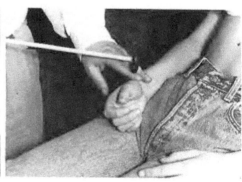

Figure 56c. Elicit supinator jerk on both sides

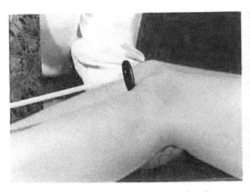

Figure 56d. Elicit knee jerk on both sides

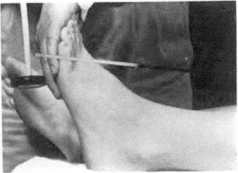

Figure 56e. Elicit ankle jerk on both sides

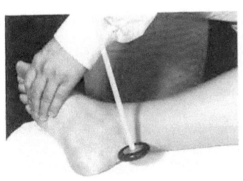

Figure 56f. (Alternative method)

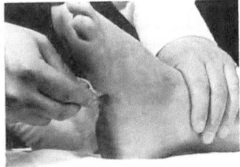

Figure 56g. Elicit plantar response on both sides

As with percussion, it takes much practise to acquire skill in the use of the patella hammer. The following points should be borne in mind:

1   Full size patella hammers are designed to be held gently at the end of the shaft between your thumb and first and second fingers (not half way down the shaft in your fist). See Figure 56h.

2   The stimulus should be applied to the tendon by letting the hammer fall through a wide, consistent arc under the influence of gravity (not by using your arm and wrist muscles as if banging in a nail). See Figure 56i.

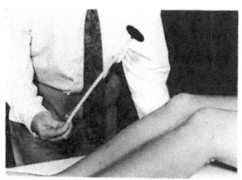
Figure 56h

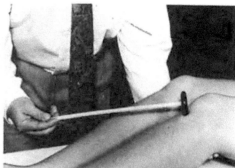
Figure 56i

3   For the purposes of general screening, one accurate hit should be enough for each reflex. As soon as you have elicited a jerk, move on to the next (instead of repeatedly hitting the same tendon).

4   If you find it hard to elicit tendon jerks in a particular patient, ask them to clench their teeth together tightly (upper limb reflexes) or pull one hand hard against the other (lower limb reflexes) as you hit the tendon. This will exaggerate the response.

5   As a general principle, it is more comfortable for the patient if you place your own fingers over the tendon being struck (see Figures above) so that the direct blow of the hammer is absorbed by you and not them. This method has the added advantage that you can sometimes feel the tendon move under your finger as the reflex is elicited.

6   The first method shown in Figure 56e for eliciting the ankle jerk is useful for elderly patients who may find it hard to abduct and externally rotate their hip joints. The foot has to be slightly dorsiflexed before trying to elicit the reflex using this method.

7   The range of normality is very wide indeed for tendon jerks. Many normal elderly people have absent ankle jerks and fit young people often have very brisk reflexes. The important thing, as in all neurological testing, is to compare sides. Markedly increased jerks on one side may suggest an UMN lesion of the opposite side (e.g. stroke). Markedly decreased jerks may suggest a LMN lesion on the same side. Cerebellar lesions may also produce diminished tendon jerks.

8   Patients with UMN lesions sometimes exhibit *clonus* (repeated alternating jerky movements) when a tendon is stretched. For example, a sharp, sustained upward push on the left foot of a right sided stroke victim may precipitate several seconds of repeated up and down movements of the foot.

9   Eliciting the plantar response involves scratching the lateral side of the sole (where the dark and the light skin meet) with the sharp end of a patella hammer or a car key upwards and then medially across the MTP joints. The first movement of the toes is the one that counts and may occur after only a centimetre or two of scratching. If the toes flex downwards, this is a normal plantar response. If the big toe moves upwards and the other toes spread out, this is abnormal and is referred to as an extensor plantar response. (Extensor plantar responses are normal in babies up to six months old). An upgoing plantar response suggests an upper motor neurone lesion of the opposite side.

PROCEDURE:
Test vibration sense in the feet

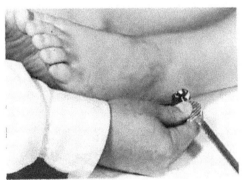

Figure 57

Hints and tips
Hold a vibrating tuning fork against the patient's sternum so that they can clearly feel the buzzing sensation. Then hold it against the external malleoli and ask if the buzzing is still felt clearly on both sides (Figure 57).

Decreased vibration sense is quite common in the elderly. It may also suggest dorsal column sensory loss (e.g. in diabetes).

PROCEDURE:

Test position sense in the feet

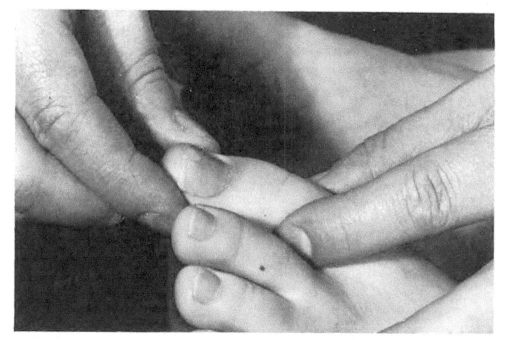

Figure 58

Hints and tips

Take hold of the sides of a big toe between your thumb and index finger, keeping the other toes out of the way with your other hand (see Figure 58). Then move the big toe up and down and ask the patient, with their eyes closed, to tell you every time they feel the toe move and in what direction (up or down). See how small a movement can be detected.

Repeat on the other side.

Dorsal column sensory loss will cause a loss of position sense.

PROCEDURE:
Briefly test sensitivity to light touch and pinprick (Figure 59)

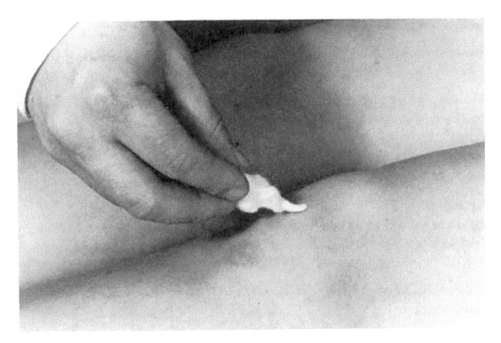

Figure 59

Hints and tips

Briefly test sensitivity first to light touch and then to pinprick over a selection of dermatomes (lower limbs, upper limbs and anterior trunk – see section on dermatomes at the end of Part 2.4) using a wisp of cotton wool and a sterile disposable pin. Compare sides as you go.

Ask the patient to close their eyes and say 'yes' when they feel the touch of the cotton wool or 'sharp' when they feel the touch of the pin.

If you find a definite area of sensory loss, try to map out its upper and lower boundaries.

Do not spend too long on these tests otherwise you and your patient will get confused.

PROCEDURE:
Perform Romberg test

Hints and tips
Ask the patient to stand with their feet together and then ask them to close their eyes and see if they remain steady.

If they start to fall, it suggests a problem with position sense and thus dorsal column sensory loss (e.g. tabes dorsalis of syphilis).

Some healthy elderly people also 'fail' this test. Always stand close enough to support your patient should they start to fall.

PROCEDURE:
Watch the patient walk

Hints and tips
Ask the patient to walk to and fro across the room and look for unusual gait. You should, in fact, have observed their walk when they first entered your consulting room.

People with Parkinson's disease walk slowly with small shuffling steps and a bent posture.

People with cerebellar lesions walk with their feet wide apart as they try to maintain their balance.

People who have had a unilateral stroke have to swing the affected leg out in a circle with each forward step to avoid scraping their toes on the ground. This is because spasticity of the lower limbs produces extension at all joints so the foot is plantar flexed.

People who have lost sensation in their feet take high steps and tend to slap their feet down on the floor.

Interpreting the results of an examination of the nervous system is easier if you have a basic understanding of dermatomes and myotomes and know the nerve roots involved in the various tendon reflexes.

The following tables may be useful as an *aide-mémoire*:

Dermatomes

The area of skin supplied by a single spinal nerve (and thus by a single segment of the spinal cord) is called a *dermatome*.

On the trunk there is considerable overlap between adjacent dermatomes.

The rather strange arrangement of dermatomes in the limbs results from changes that take place as the limbs grow outward from the body wall during embryological development.

The following table represents a minimum basic knowledge of dermatome 'levels':

TABLE 2

C4	Tip of shoulder
C5	Lateral aspect of elbow
C6	Thumb
C7	Middle finger
C8	Little finger
T3	Axilla
T8	Costal margin
T10	Umbilicus
T12	Pubis
L3	Knee
L5	Big toe
S1	Little toe

Myotomes

Skeletal muscle also receives a segmental innervation, but most muscles are innervated by two, three or four spinal nerves. Thus the concept of myotomes (muscles supplied by particular combinations of spinal nerves) is clinically useful in localizing lesions in the motor (efferent) nervous system to approximate levels in the spinal cord.

The following table lists the muscles tested routinely in clinical examination together with their segmental and specific innervation:

TABLE 3

Shoulder abduction:	Deltoid	C5 (axillary nerve)
Elbow flexion:	Biceps	C5/6 (musculocutaneous nerve)
Wrist extension:	Long extensors	C6/7 (radial/post. interosseous n.)
Hand grip:	Intrinsic hand muscles	C8/T1 (ulnar/median n.)
Spread fingers:	Intrinsic hand muscles	Ulnar nerve
Opposed little finger and thumb:	Opponens pollicis	Median nerve
Hip flexion:	Iliopsoas	L2/3 (femoral nerve)
Knee flexion:	Hamstrings	L5/S1 (sciatic nerve)
Knee extension:	Quadriceps	L3/4 (femoral nerve)
Foot dorsiflex:	Tibialis anterior	L4/5 (deep peroneal nerve)
Foot plantarflex:	Gastrocnemius/Soleus	S1/2 (post. tibial nerve)

Tendon Reflexes

TABLE 4

Biceps	C5/6
Supinator	C6
Triceps	C7/8
Patellar tendon	L3/4
Achilles tendon	S1/2
Plantar reflex	L5–S2

Recording the Results of your Examination

Record your findings once the examination is completed

- Higher functions
- Cranial nerves II to XII
- Pupils equal size and reacting to light and accommodation (PERLA)
- Fundi
- Upper limb tone/power/co-ordination

- Lower limb tone/power/co-ordination
- Reflexes (biceps, supinator, triceps, knee, ankle, plantar) left and right
- Sensory testing (vibration, position sense, light touch, pinprick)

In more or less standard medical shorthand, entry in the notes for a person with a normal nervous system might read:

Higher functions NAD
CN II–XII: NAD
PERLA
Fundi: NAD
Tone/power/co-ordination: normal upper/lower

Reflexes	B	S	T	K	A	PLANTAR
Left	+	+	+	+	+	⬎
Right	+	+	+	+	+	⬎
Sensory:	NAD					

2.5 EXAMINING THE JOINTS

Basic Routine

Detailed assessment of joint function is a skilled procedure requiring much practice. However, the underlying principles are simple:

- Does each joint look normal?
- Does each joint feel normal?
- Can the patient move each joint through a full range of movement without pain?
- Is the range of active movement (the patient moving the joint) more or less the same as the range of passive movement (you moving the joint for them)?

The following scheme is only intended as an introductory screening and does not include specific tests for ligament damage. I suggest you examine the appendicular joints first and then look for spinal deformity, tenderness over each vertebra and restriction of spinal movements afterwards.

- General observation (posture, walk, spinal deformity, height, shape and size of limbs and skull, muscle wasting).
- Look at each joint in turn comparing left with right. Is there any swelling or deformity?
- Feel each joint in turn comparing left with right. Is there tenderness, heat or swelling? (For the spine, a firm tap with the side of a closed fist over each palpable vertebra in turn should elicit any spinal tenderness).
- Ask the patient to move each joint in turn (see below for normal ranges of movement) comparing left with right. Is the range of active movement normal? Is the movement painful?
- Move each joint yourself with the patient relaxed, comparing left with right. Is the range of passive movement similar to the active range? Is there pain? Can you feel any unusual crunching sensations as you move the joint with one hand whilst feeling over it with the other?

The following pictures demonstrate the normal range of movement (in relation to standard reference positions) for each joint in turn.

Shoulder

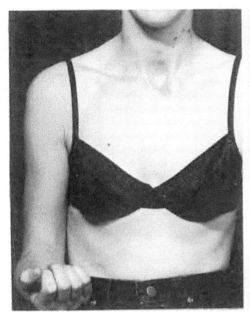

Figure 60. Neutral

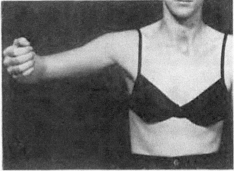

Figure 62. 90 degrees abduction
(gleno-humeral)

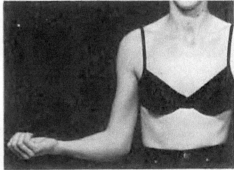

Figure 63. 60 degrees external rotation

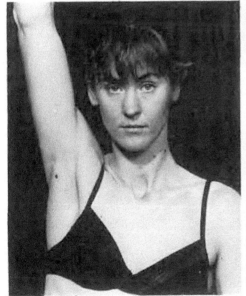

Figure 61. 180 degrees abduction

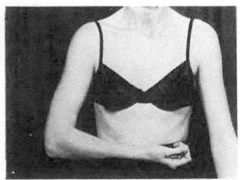

Figure 64. 90 degrees internal rotation

Elbow

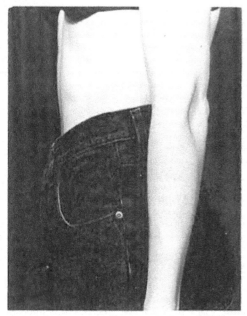

Figure 65. Neutral

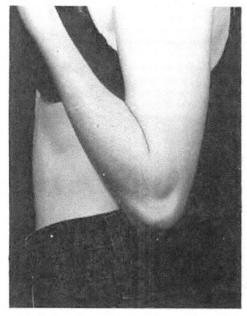

Figure 66. 150 degrees flexion

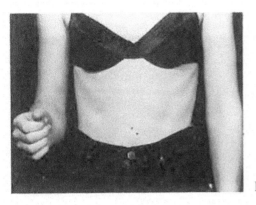

Figure 67. Neutral

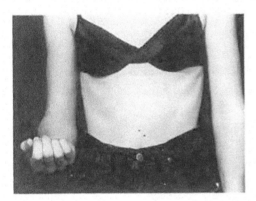

Figure 68. 90 degrees supination

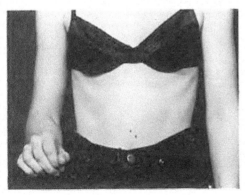

Figure 69. 80 degrees pronation

Wrist

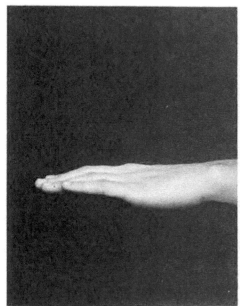

Figure 70. Neutral

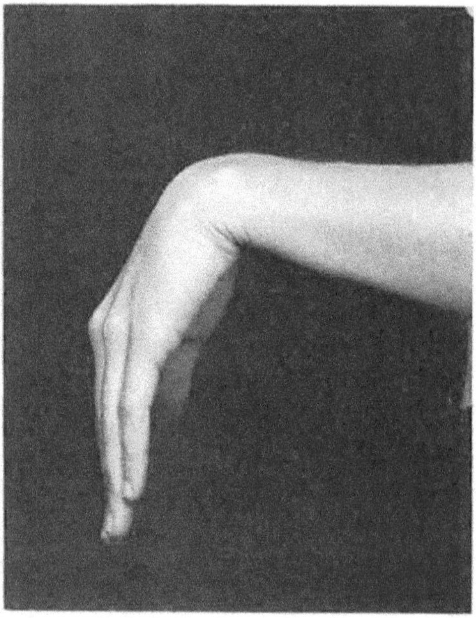

Figure 71. 75 degrees flexion

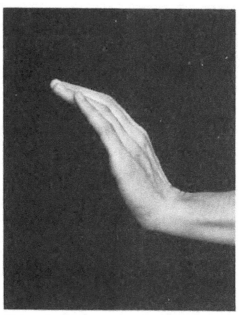

Figure 72. 70 degrees extension

Hip

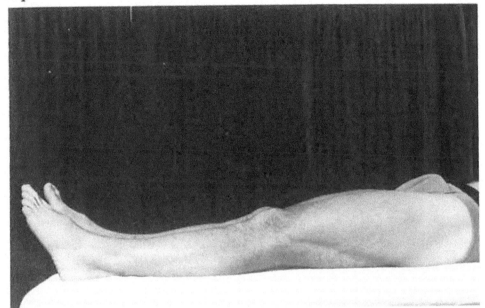

Figure 73. Neutral

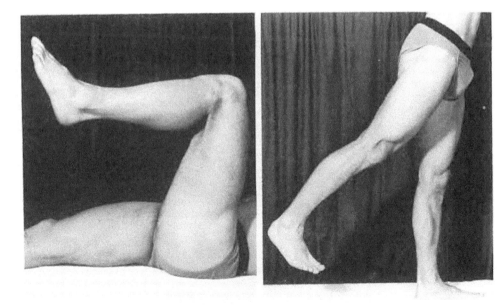

Figure 74. 115 degrees flexion   Figure 75. 30 degrees extension

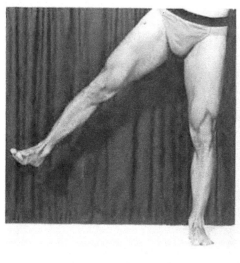

Figure 76. 50 degrees abduction

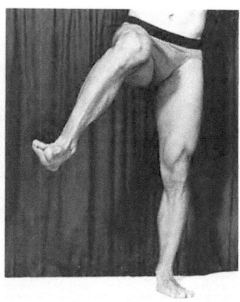

Figure 77. 45 degrees internal rotation

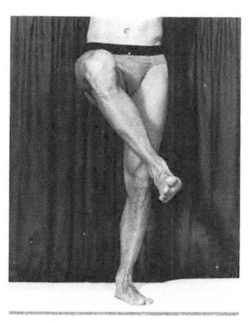

Figure 78. 45 degrees external rotation

Knee

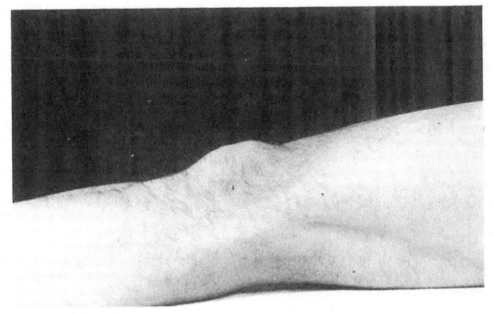

Figure 79. Neutral

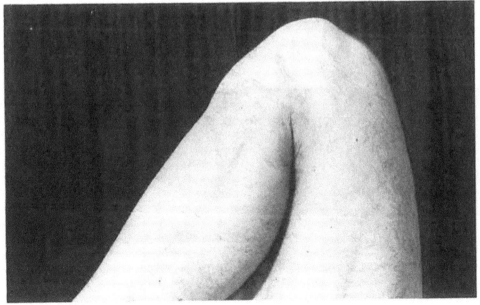

Figure 80. 135 degrees flexion (Note: 5 degrees hyperextension is also possible)

Ankle

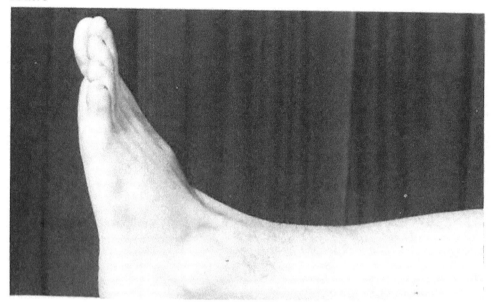

Figure 81. Neutral

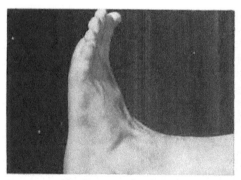

Figure 82. 30 degrees dorsiflexion

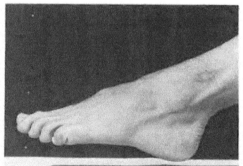

Figure 83. 50 degrees plantarflexion

Spinal Movements

Cervical

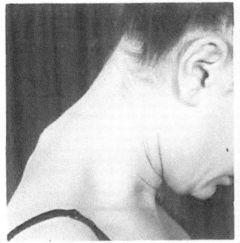

Figure 84. Flexion

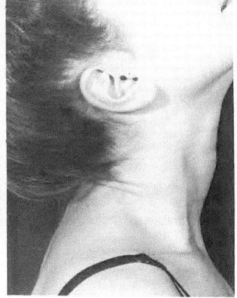

Figure 85. Extension

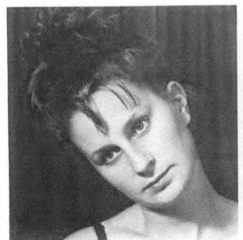

Figure 86. Lateral

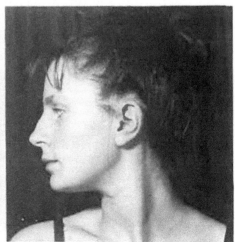

Figure 87. Rotation

Thoracic

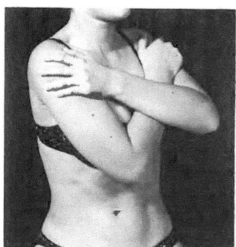

Figure 88. Rotation

Lumbar

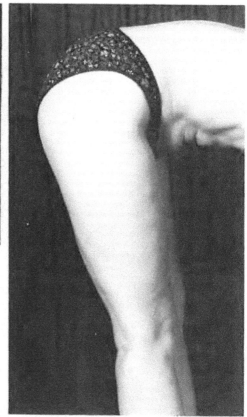

Figure 89. Flexion

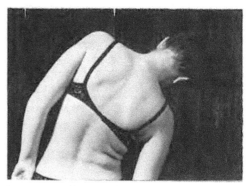

Figure 90. Sidebending

Note 1: Effusions

If a joint is swollen because fluid has collected in or around it, the normal 'dimples' around the joint are often filled out and distorted and the joint feels 'squishy' on palpation. It may be possible to see or feel fluid moving around the joint as you palpate, e.g. if you press gently on a lateral swelling of a swollen knee joint you may see the fluid shift, causing a bulge to appear for a moment on the medial side.

The technical name for a collection of fluid around a joint is an **effusion**. The jargon for 'squishy' is fluctuant. Effusions around the knee may cause the patella to 'float' free of the underlying joint. If you press down on such a patella, you may elicit the sensation of it moving downwards through a viscous fluid and coming to rest with a clunk on the underlying bone. This is known as a patellar tap and is looked for in the following way:

Milk the fluid from above and below the knee into the middle of the joint with both hands (Figure 91).

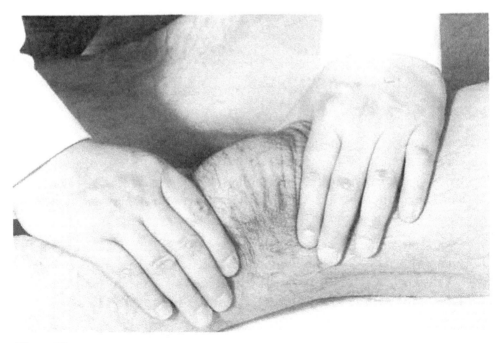

Figure 91

Use the forefinger of one hand to push down firmly on the patella and see if it moves down and hits the underlying bone with a definite tap or clunk (Figure 92).

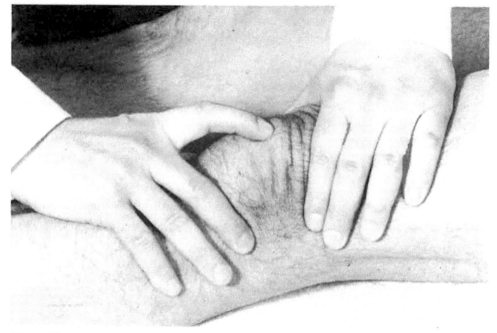

Figure 92

Note 2: Straight leg raising

In healthy people with reasonable joint mobility, it should be possible for you to raise each of their legs off the bed in turn and, keeping the knee straight, flex the hip joint to almost 90 degrees. However, 'straight leg raising' in a person with a prolapsed intervertebral disc affecting lower lumbar/upper sacral nerve roots causes back pain which may radiate down the leg.

One way of performing the normal straight leg raising test is to lift the leg off the couch with the knee straight until the patient just feels pain in their back (+/– sciatica). The leg is then lowered a few degrees and the foot dorsiflexed. This action stretches the sciatic nerve and thus brings the pain on again.

This test is useful in distinguishing the pain of 'tight hamstrings' or an arthritic hip from the pain of a prolapsed intervertebral disc.

Recording the Results of your Examination

Once you have recorded details of any general observations (noting in particular whether joint problems are affecting single or multiple joints and whether multiple joint problems are symmetrical or asymmetrical), it is a matter of personal taste how you record the rest of the information. Drawings and diagrams are particularly useful and some practitioners have standard pictures included on their pre-printed case history sheets on which to record their findings.

However, stick figure drawings are perfectly acceptable.

2.6 THE MENTAL STATE EXAMINATION

Assessment of the mental state is a specialist skill best learnt in the practical situation under the guidance of an experienced professional. However, it is important for all practitioners to have some system for assessing a patient's mental processes as objectively as possible and preferably in a way that does not rely entirely on the patient's co-operation.

The following scheme is not sufficient to allow the specific diagnosis of psychiatric illness but should at least enable the practitioner to decide whether mental disorder is a realistic possibility. In particular, I believe it is important for every practitioner to be able to recognize the presence of organic brain dysfunction (since this may be treatable).

Thus, whether you routinely make an assessment of the mental state of your patients or not, you must make some judgement about their cognitive ability, (i.e. do they know who they are and where they are, and can they remember events from the recent and distant past as well as anyone else would in comparable circumstances?). If they cannot, they may have serious but potentially treatable organic brain pathology and must be referred for further investigation.

Taking a normal history and performing routine physical examination will usually provide more than enough information for a simple assessment of the mental state and the information gained can be summarized and recorded under the following headings:

NON-VERBAL BEHAVIOUR
SOCIAL MANNER
NON-VERBAL EXPRESSION OF MOOD
SPEECH (which is taken to be a reflection of underlying thought processes)
COGNITIVE ABILITY (level of consciousness, orientation, memory and concentration)

The following list outlines what to look for under each heading:

Non-verbal behaviour

Dress:
Is it clean?
Is it unusually drab or colourful?
Are there any unusual adornments or accessories?

Walk:
Fast or slow
Odd

Motor activity:
Tics
Mannerisms

Social manner

Aggressive
Withdrawn
Friendly
Open

Non-verbal expression of mood

Sad
Anxious
Depressed
Cheerful
Elated
Angry

Speech

Form of speech:
Rate
Quantity
Volume
Tone
Grammar
Unusual associations or changes of topic

Content of speech:
Delusions
Hallucinations
Expressions of mood disturbance, anxieties, obsessions or compulsions

Cognitive function

Level of consciousness:
Awake and alert
Irritable
Drowsy
Asleep but rousable
Asleep and rousable only with strong stimuli (e.g. pain)
Asleep, non-rousable but reacting to painful stimuli by reflex withdrawal
Dead

Orientation:
Space
Time
Person

Memory:
Recent
Past

Concentration

Cognitive function can be assessed by using the following simple questions:

What is your name?
How old are you?
What is your address?
What day is it?
What year is it?
Where is this place we are in now?
Who am I?
What year did ... (any question appropriate to the patient's age and background)
Who is the Prime Minister at the moment?
Can you subtract seven from 100 in your head?
Subtract seven from the answer
And again ...
And again ...

Most of these questions (or equivalents) can be asked, if necessary, as part of routine history taking.

Recording the Results of your Examination

A mental state examination should be recorded under the five headings:

Non-verbal behaviour
Social manner
Non-verbal expression of mood
Speech
Cognitive ability

TOPICS OF SPECIAL INTEREST

3.1 LUMPS IN THE SKIN AND SUBCUTANEOUS TISSUES

Examining Lumps

Examining lumps is an important part of primary care and the statement 'I've had this thing here for a few days/weeks/months/years and I was just wondering whether it was anything to worry about' is familiar to all practitioners. Often, the subtext is 'do you think this lump is cancerous?'.

You will already have learnt that malignant lumps are usually distinguishable from their benign cousins by rapid growth, irregular shape, hard texture, fixity to surrounding tissue and a tendency to produce systemic disturbance such as malaise and weight loss. Malignant growths also tend to spread to other sites, e.g. bone and liver.

However, when confronted with a lump in the clinical situation, the tendency is to look at it, poke it a bit and still wonder what it is; so a systematic approach is needed to make sure that malignant lumps are not missed, that inflammatory lumps are distinguished from neoplastic lumps and that all lumps are managed appropriately.

I suggest that you get into the habit of assessing the following attributes of any lump that you come across:

Position	Consistency
Size	Mobility
Shape	Relationship to surrounding tissues
Number	Tenderness
Depth	Colour of underlying skin
Surface contour	Any relevant concurrent symptoms or signs

It may also be helpful to hold a torch against one side of the lump and see if it 'transilluminates' (lets light through). Solid lumps do not, fluid filled lumps do. You should also listen over the lump with a stethoscope in case it is very vascular, in which case you will hear a soft whooshing noise (bruit).

Determining the depth of a lump below the surface can be tricky. The key is to think anatomically as you feel. Lumps confined entirely to the skin will move around as you move the skin around, independent of underlying structures. Lumps within a muscle will become immobile and fixed if that muscle is tensed. Lumps below the muscle layer will be palpable as long as the overlying muscles are relaxed but will seem to disappear when they are contracted.

TABLE 5

TYPES OF SKIN LUMP

Papillomas – benign skin tags

Warts – benign neoplasms caused by the wart virus

Seborrhoeic warts – benign, slow growing patches of slightly pigmented, raised skin common in the elderly

Mole – benign overgrowth of melanin-producing cells

Malignant melanoma – malignant tumour of melanin-producing cells

Haemangiomas – tumours of vascular tissue

Pyogenic granulomas – overgrowth of granulation tissue covered with epithelium at the site of a healed wound

Keratoacanthoma – benign overgrowth of a sebaceous gland

Keloid – gross hypertrophy of scar tissue

Solar keratosis – thickened, darkened patches of sun-damaged skin

Basal cell carcinoma – also called rodent ulcer. Cancer of basal cells of epidermis, usually seen on the face

Squamous cell carcinoma – more aggressive form of epidermal cell cancer related to sun damage and chemical exposure

Boils – infection of hair follicle showing the classical signs of inflammation. A group of confluent boils is called a carbuncle

TABLE 6

TYPES OF SUBCUTANEOUS LUMP

Lipomas – soft, lobulated, mobile, benign tumours of fat cells

Sebaceous cyst – distended sebaceous gland caused by blockage of its opening. They often have what appears to be a little hole or depression in the middle

Ganglion – jelly filled lumps of degenerate fibrous tissue often found in extensor tendon sheaths near joints

Neurofibromas – benign tumours of nervous tissue. Multiple neurofibromatosis is an inherited condition (von Recklinghausen's disease) characterized by nerve tumours, skin tags and patches of skin discolouration known as *café-au-lait* patches

Abscess – a collection of pus surrounded by granulation tissue

It is beyond the scope of this book to discuss any of these conditions further. You may have seen some of them already and clear pictures of the others can be found in most large textbooks of medicine and pathology.

Moreover, it can take years of specialist clinical experience before sure differentiation between types of skin lump becomes second nature and you may never see some of the conditions listed above in practice. The important thing, therefore, is to examine every skin lump you see in a thorough and systematic way. You must then assess its significance in the context of the whole clinical picture. If you are left with even the slightest suspicion of malignant change or severe infection, **seek expert help and advice.**

3.2 LUMPS IN THE NECK

Introduction

There are so many possible causes of a lump in the neck that the topic has become one of perennial fascination for medical students, their teachers and examiners. This sometimes obscures the fact that there are only two common causes of neck swellings: **enlarged lymph nodes** and an **enlarged thyroid gland.** The most important feature distinguishing thyroid swellings from other lumps is that thyroid swellings move up and down on swallowing. Thus the everyday clinical problem of a lump in the neck is unlikely to be as complicated as the classification outlined on page 128 makes it look.

For, as with lumps elsewhere, your objectives are:

1   To notice that there is a lump in the first place
2   To examine each lump carefully and systematically as described in Part 3.1
3   To record your findings clearly
4   To seek further help and advice if you do not know what the lump is, or are unsure about its significance

You will remember from your study of anatomy that the side of the neck can be regarded as being divided into two triangles, the **anterior triangle** and the **posterior triangle**. The dividing line between the two is the sternomastoid muscle. Neck swellings are usually described as being (i) in the midline; (ii) in the anterior triangle, or (iii) in the posterior triangle.

Looking for Cervical Lymphadenopathy (swollen lymph nodes in the neck)

Broadly speaking, lymph nodes enlarge in response to one of four pathological processes:

- Infection (local or generalized)
- Metastatic malignancy
- Primary malignancy (such as Hodgkin's disease)
- Sarcoidosis

It does not really matter how you examine for cervical lymphadenopathy (some people always examine the neck from behind, others from in front) but you should do it the same way each time. You should also realize that the common places to find swollen lymph nodes are

- under the jaw
- along the anterior border of the sternomastoid
- in the supraclavicular fossa
- along the anterior border of trapezius
- under the occiput (e.g. in children with German measles)

Thus a logical scheme for examining the neck for swollen lymph glands would be:

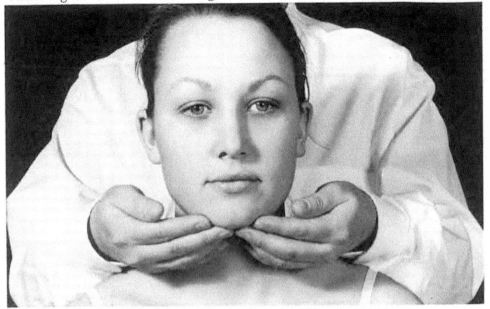

- Start with the fingers of both hands feeling underneath the jaw at the front (Figure 93).

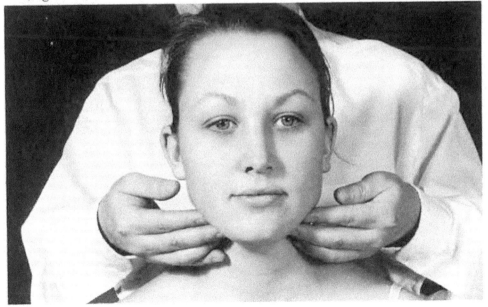

- Work backwards towards the angle of the jaw on each side (Figure 94)...

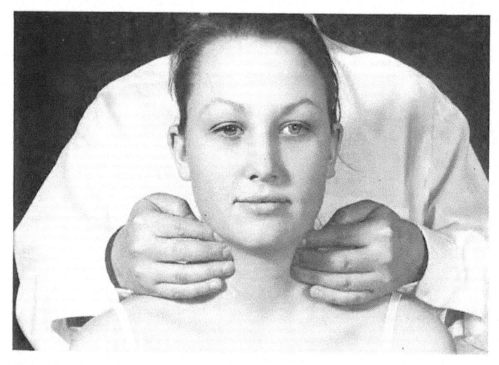

- and then down the anterior border of the sternomastoid (Figure 95).

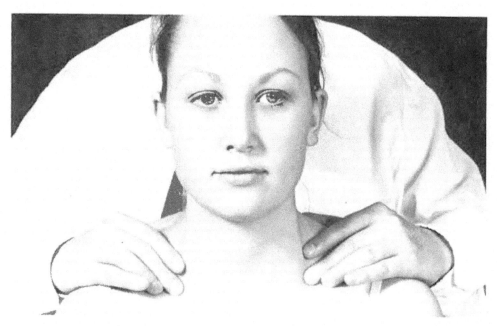

- Feel outwards along the supraclavicular fossa (Figure 96)...

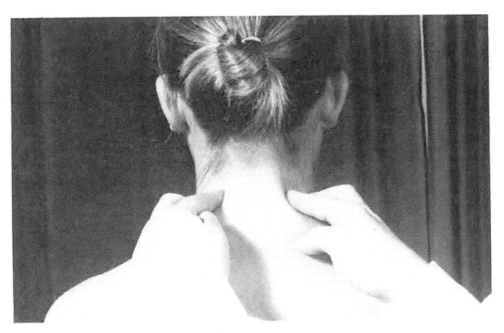

- and then up the anterior edge of the trapezius (Figure 97).

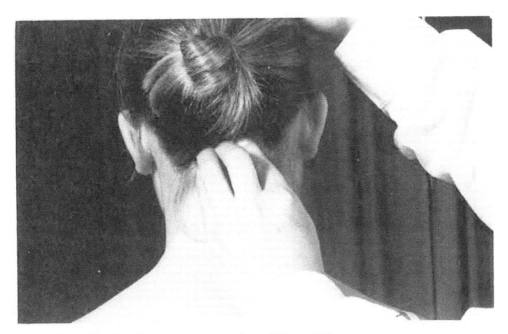

- Finish off by feeling under the occiput (Figure 98).

If you find a lump, remember to assess it in all the ways mentioned in Part 3.1.

You will see practitioners use all sorts of ways of moving their fingers when feeling for lymph nodes: one of the favourites is to drag the fingers slightly as they 'walk up and down the neck'. This makes any enlarged nodes obvious as they slip under the fingers.

Note: It is quite common for people who have had a lymph node 'come up' in response to some infection or other to find that, instead of going away when they are well, it shrinks into a firm, pea-like entity which is fun to fiddle with. These hardly ever disappear but are not significant.

Looking for an Enlarged Thyroid

As you know, thyroid swellings are often associated with abnormal levels of thyroid hormone in the blood and it is very important before you start to feel for an enlarged gland to observe the patient's general state.

A patient with an overactive thyroid (thyrotoxicosis) may be agitated with sweaty hands, a fine hand tremor and a fast heartbeat. Their eyes may look abnormal and show signs of lid retraction (sclera visible between the top of the iris and the upper lid) or exophthalmos (sclera visible above and below the iris with eye pushed forward and reddened).

A patient with an underactive thyroid may look tired and lethargic with puffy, dry skin, coarse hair, cold hands and a hoarse voice.

Your objectives in examining the thyroid gland are to determine:

- Is the gland swollen?
- If it is, is it swollen by a single lump, by several lumps or by diffuse enlargement?
- Are there any signs of thyroid hormone level abnormality?

A suggested routine for examining the thyroid is:

- Assess the general state of the patient and look carefully at the eyes

- Look carefully at the neck from the front, looking for swelling or asymmetry (Figure 99).

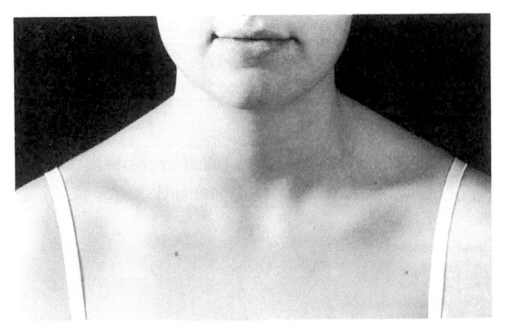

Figure 99

- Hand the patient a glass of water; look at the surface of the water to see if there is any fine, rapid tremor (indicating thyrotoxicosis).
- Ask the patient to swallow and look to see if any swelling you may have noticed moves upwards when they do.
- Stand behind the patient and feel over the thyroid with your hands flat and fingers straight (Figure 100). If you feel a lump, ask the patient to swallow again and see if it moves upwards.

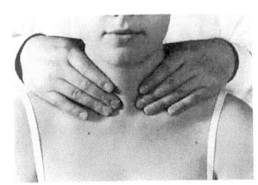

Figure 100

- If you are sure you have found a swelling, try to determine its characteristics as usual and record the information carefully. It may be useful to percuss over the gland from the front to try to determine how far below the sternum it goes. If you listen over an enlarged thyroid with a stethoscope, you may hear a bruit.

Simplified Classification of Lumps in the Neck (based on their position)

Superficial (see Part 3.1):
- Sebaceous cysts
- Lipomas
- Boils and carbuncles
- Neurofibroma

Deep and more or less midline:
- Thyroglossal cyst (developmental abnormality seen as a round, firm midline swelling that move upwards when the owner protrudes their tongue)
- Pharyngeal pouch (a herniation of the pharyngeal mucosa through a weakness in the posterior pharyngeal muscles. The soft lump usually appears to the left of the midline, for some reason. It can be the cause of irritating and noisy food regurgitation)
- Cancer of the trachea, larynx or oesophagus

Deep and lateral:
- Lymph nodes
- Thyroid swellings
- Swollen salivary gland (e.g. infection, tumour or obstruction of gland outlet by a stone or stricture)
- Branchial cyst (soft, deep swelling found in young people at the angle of the jaw, spreading into the anterior triangle. Caused by developmental abnormality)

- Sternomastoid tumour (a lump of scar tissue within the sternomastoid muscle which may cause postural problems with the neck. Some people think they result from birth trauma)
- Cervical rib (if this extra rib presses on the T1 nerve root it will cause pins and needles/numbness over the T1 dermatome. It may also distort the course of the subclavian artery. This in turn may produce a pulsing lump palpable just above the clavicle)
- Cystic Hygroma (seen in babies and caused by a failure of development of lymph vessels. Forms a soft, deep swelling in the posterior triangle)
- Carotid body tumour (smooth, painless and usually benign tumour of carotid body chemoreceptor cells that causes a lump in the carotid artery at about the level of the top of the thyroid cartilage in middle-aged adults. Very, very rare (but interesting none the less))

3.3 LUMPS IN THE GROIN

Introduction

The word **hernia** means the protrusion of some or all of a body part out of its normal place through a gap in the wall of its surrounding cavity. The commonest external hernias are found in the groin – inguinal hernias – but external hernias occur in many sites, e.g. through and around the umbilicus, through old operation scars, etc.

The common causes of a lump in the groin are lymph nodes and inguinal hernias. In order to tell the difference when examining someone complaining of a lump in the groin, you need to remember the following anatomical facts:

- The inguinal ligament runs from the anterior superior iliac spine to the pubic tubercle
- The pubic tubercles are about 2cm away from the midline on the top edge of the pubic bones
- The inguinal canal runs from the internal inguinal ring to the external inguinal ring

- The internal ring lies about 1.5cm above the inguinal ligament at the mid-inguinal point, i.e. halfway along an imaginary line joining the ASIS to the pubic symphysis
- The external ring lies about 1cm above and *medial* to the pubic tubercle
- The femoral canal opens below and *lateral* to the pubic tubercle

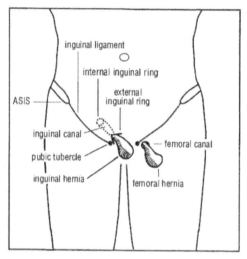

Diagram 2

You should also remember the following basic facts about hernias:

- They emerge through weak spots in the abdominal musculature (e.g. the inguinal rings)
- Weak spots in abdominal musculature can be caused by surgery or trauma
- Weak spots in abdominal musculature are exaggerated by raised intra-abdominal pressure from coughing (e.g. smokers), straining (e.g. constipation) or abdominal distension (e.g. someone with ascites)
- Most hernias can be 'put back' (reduced) by lying down or by pressing on them (hernias that won't reduce may need urgent attention)
- Hernias expand upwards and outwards when their owners cough, i.e. they have an expansile cough impulse

Remember also that:

Indirect inguinal hernias come out of the internal inguinal ring, pass down and medially via the inguinal canal, come out of the external inguinal ring passing above and medial to the pubic tubercle and may then pass into the scrotum (in males). By implication, when an indirect inguinal hernia is reduced, if you keep your fingers pressed over the internal inguinal ring, the hernia will not come out again even if the patient coughs.

Direct inguinal hernias 'ignore' the internal inguinal ring and push out directly forwards through the external ring. They cannot, therefore, be controlled by pressure over the internal ring.

Femoral hernias are swellings that emerge through the femoral canal. The neck of a femoral hernia is thus always below and lateral to the pubic tubercle, unlike inguinal hernias whose necks are always above and medial to the pubic tubercle.

Examining Lumps in the Groin

- With the patient lying down and the groin creases exposed, look at the lower abdomen and remind yourself of the basic anatomy of the region.
- Ask the patient to turn their head away from you and cough. Look for an abnormal expansile bulge appearing somewhere near the groin crease.
- Place your hands flat over the inguinal ligaments, fingers pointing downwards and medially towards the pubic symphysis. Ask the patient to cough again; is there an expansile swelling? (Figure 101).

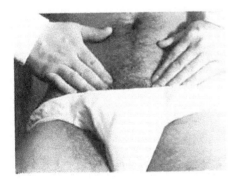

Figure 101

- If you do suspect a hernia, stand the patient up and, kneeling so that your head is at the same height as the groin crease, repeat your observation and palpation, one side at a time, as the patient coughs.

- If you find a hernia, put it back gently ('reduce it') or ask the patient to put it back and see if it can be 'controlled' by pressure over the internal inguinal ring.
- If there is no evidence of hernia, briefly palpate the inguinal region for other lumps (e.g. lymph nodes).

Other Possible Causes of a Lump in the Groin

Remember, the only really common causes of lumps in the groin are inguinal hernias and swollen lymph nodes.

Apart from these, the following are sometimes seen:

- Femoral hernia (see above)
- Saphena varix (a varicosity of the long saphenous vein that appears below the inguinal ligament and disappears when the leg is lifted up with the patient lying down)
- Femoral aneurysm (a pulsing lump below the inguinal ligament usually associated with severe atherosclerosis)
- Hydrocoele of the spermatic cord (a tense, cystic swelling that may occur anywhere along the length of the spermatic cord and which moves downwards when the testis on that side is pulled downwards)
- Undescended or ectopic testis (check to see if both testes are in the scrotum)

3.4 LUMPS IN THE BREAST

Introduction

Brief examination of the breasts can be carried out at any convenient time during a routine physical examination.

There are four major indicators of breast disease:

- Lumps

- Nipple retraction
- Nipple discharge
- Pain

All of these may reflect underlying malignancy. All may also be caused by treatable inflammatory or benign neoplastic conditions.

Take account of the phase of the menstrual cycle when examining breasts. Remember that breast cancer is a relatively common disease and that it also occurs in men (approximately 1 per cent).

Examining the Breasts

- Sit your patient facing you on the side of the couch and look carefully at breasts for any asymmetry, lumps, retracted nipples or changes in skin texture in one part of a breast (Figure 102).

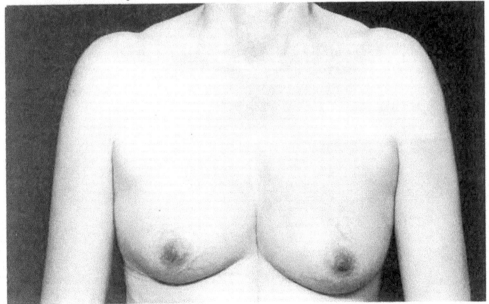

Figure 102

- Ask the patient to slowly raise their arms above their head (Figure 103) and look to see if any asymmetry or unusual skin creasing appears (suggesting tethering of the skin by an underlying malignancy).

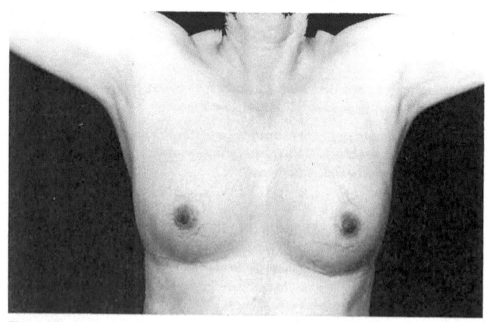

Figure 103

- Lie the patient nearly flat and ask them to put the arm on the side of the breast you are going to examine over their head and lean away from that side until the breast is arranged symmetrically over the chest wall (Figure 104).

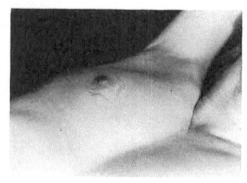

Figure 104

- Feel each quadrant of the breast with your hand flat. (Figure 105).
- If you find a lump, test its mobility, etc, as for any other lump.
- Examine the other breast.

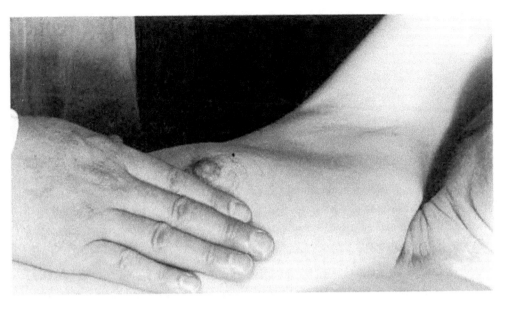

Figure 105

If you feel a suspicious lump in either breast:

- Feel for swollen lymph nodes on the four sides of each armpit (anterior wall, posterior wall, medial wall, lateral wall). It helps if you support your patient's arm with your free hand while you are doing this so that the muscles surrounding the armpit are relaxed. You should feel as high up into the axilla as possible when looking for swollen lymph nodes (Figure 106).
- Feel for swollen lymph nodes in the supraclavicular fossae.
- Feel to see if there is any liver enlargement (see Part 2.3).

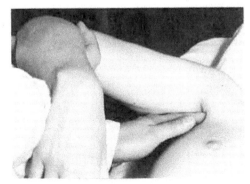

Figure 106

3.5 BLOOD PRESSURE MEASUREMENT

General Principles

A fabric cuff containing an inflatable rubber bag attached to a pressure measurement gauge is wrapped around the upper arm and inflated until the flow of blood through the brachial artery is entirely obstructed.

The pressure in the cuff is then reduced until the pressure in the artery under the cuff is just enough to open the artery momentarily and force some blood through. This can be heard as a knocking sound through a stethoscope placed over the brachial artery.

The measured pressure at which knocking sounds are first heard is equal to the systolic pressure (i.e. the maximum pressure generated by the heart in the cardiac cycle).

If the pressure in the cuff is decreased further, a point will be reached where the knocking sounds disappear (or suddenly go very quiet). The measurement at this moment represents diastolic pressure (the lowest level to which the blood pressure drops during the cardiac cycle). Blood flow through a normal unobstructed artery cannot be heard though a stethoscope, so when the sounds disappear, the pressure in the artery must be just enough to overcome the pressure from the cuff throughout the cardiac cycle.

Basic Sequence for Blood Pressure Measurement

The technique of blood pressure measurement must be learnt in a practical setting and should be practised as often as possible.

The following sequence is intended simply as an *aide-mémoire*:

- Choose correct sized cuff for patient.
- 'Unplug' the cuff tubing from machine (mercury column only).
- Wrap the cuff firmly around upper arm leaving antecubital fossa unobstructed by cuff or tubing (Figure 107).

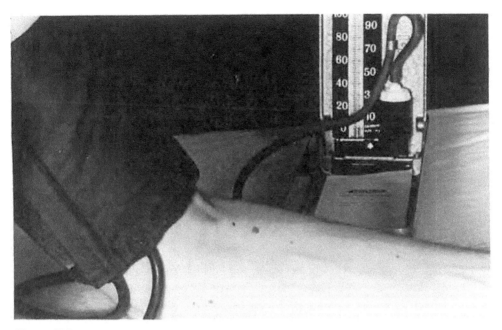

Figure 107

- Reconnect cuff tubing to machine.
- Fiddle with pressure release valve knob so that you know which way is open and which way is closed.
- Palpate the radial pulse and pump up the cuff until the pulse just disappears. This gives you a rough idea of the systolic pressure and avoids the need to pump the cuff up any higher than necessary when using the stethoscope.

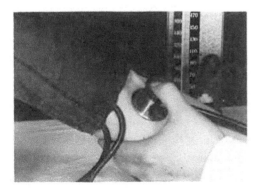

Figure 108

- Place the diaphragm of the stethoscope over the brachial artery in antecubital fossa while supporting the patient's arm straight with your fingers under their elbow and with your thumb holding the stethoscope in place (Figure 108).
- Pump up the cuff until the dial/mercury column reads about 20mmHg higher than your rough estimate of systolic pressure.
- Release the pressure in the cuff fairly slowly and note the systolic pressure (sounds appear) and the diastolic pressure (sounds disappear).

Notes

1   Do not keep the cuff inflated any longer than necessary. Emergency release of pressure can be achieved by disconnecting the tubing from the machine.

2   Mercury manometers are generally regarded as more reliable than machines with dials. Nevertheless, no BP measurement should be regarded as accurate to within more than 5mm of mercury (so a measurement of 163/84 should be recorded as 165/85).

3   If using a mercury column, remember to have the measuring scale on the machine at the same level as your eye (or vice versa) to avoid parallax errors.

4   Small cuffs on big people cause you to overestimate blood pressure; big cuffs on small people (e.g. children) cause you to underestimate blood pressure.

3.6 USE OF THE OPHTHALMOSCOPE AND AURISCOPE

The Ophthalmoscope

Ophthalmoscopic examination of the eye is an important (though often neglected) part of the examination of the cardiovascular and nervous systems. It provides the practitioner with a unique opportunity to examine living nerves and blood vessels directly. Students often find their first attempts at fundoscopy frustrating and unproductive and mastering the ophthalmoscope takes much practice. The following hints will hopefully enable you to get the most out of your practical training.

Which instrument to buy

As with all medical equipment, it usually pays in the long run to buy the best instrument you can afford. The larger, heavier models equipped with halogen bulbs are better balanced, easier to handle and easier to see through. They will also probably last a lifetime.

Controls

In essence, the ophthalmoscope is an instrument which allows you to shine a beam of light through the pupil of the eye being examined and on to the various structures beyond. By observing the light reflected back from the eye through the viewing hole in the ophthalmoscope, you can study the appearance of the veins and arteries that run over the retina and also assess the condition of the optic nerve which forms the optic disc.

An ophthalmoscope is thus usually equipped with wheels or dials that allow you to:

- Control the intensity of the light beam; if it is too bright, it will tend to cause the pupil to contract thus restricting your view of the retina. (The slider or wheel that adjusts the intensity of the light beam usually doubles as an on/off switch.)
- Place a variety of convex and concave lenses in the path of the returning light beam thus allowing you to 'correct' for long or short sightedness in you or the patient and focus on particular structures within the patient's eye.

Expensive instruments also offer a variety of beam widths (small diameter beams can be used for small diameter pupils), beam shapes (a slit of light makes it easier to assess the concavity of the optic disc) and beam colour (green light makes blood vessels and any pathological haemorrhages that may be present stand out black against a pale background).

Moving the lens strength control wheel causes numbers (corresponding to the degree of concavity or convexity of the lens selected) to appear in a small window on the examiner's side of the instrument (Figure 109).

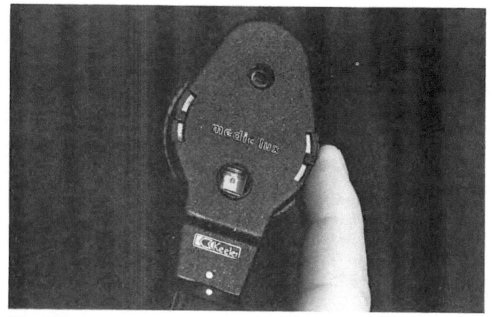

Figure 109

Simply put, black or plus numbers indicate the strength of convex lenses selected and are used to correct for long-sight in you or the patient. Red or minus numbers represent the strength of concave lenses selected and can be used to correct for short-sight. Some instruments offer a second lens system which multiplies the strength of the basic lenses by a fixed amount (convex or concave).

Examination Routine

The pictures of normal and diseased fundi seen in medical textbooks are obtained by ophthalmoscopic examination through artificially dilated pupils. Thus you should realize that you are only going to get a partial view of the retina through your ophthalmoscope since you will not be using drops to dilate the pupil.

The following routine will hopefully maximize your chances of seeing something meaningful (instead of an indistinct red blur) through your ophthalmoscope.

- If the patient wears spectacles, ask them to remove them (contact lenses are OK). It is usually easier if you remove your spectacles as well (if worn) although you may then have to set the lens selection wheel on the ophthalmoscope to a minus number to correct for your own short-sight. (Looking through the ophthalmoscope at the creases on your palm from a distance of a few centimetres and turning the lens selection wheel until the lines come into clear focus is a rough way of finding out if you need to adjust the ophthalmoscope for defects in your own vision).
- Turn off the lights/draw the curtains so that the room is reasonably dark.
- To examine the patient's right eye, hold the ophthalmoscope in your right hand and look through the aperture with your right eye. Keep your elbow close to your body and your wrist extended. Your head, arm and ophthalmoscope should then move as a single unit. The lens power selection wheel can be operated with the index finger (Figure 110).

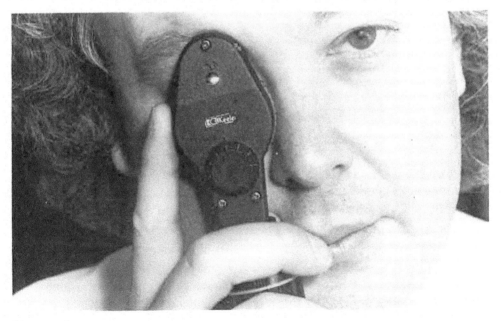

Figure 110

- Move the lens selection wheel until 0 is showing on the dial.
- Ask the patient to stare fixedly straight ahead into the distance (choose some convenient object on the far side of the room) and to try to ignore you shining a bright light into their eye.
- Keeping the instrument 20 or 30cm from the patient's eye, shine the light on to the pupil from an angle of about 15–20 degrees lateral to their line of sight and then bring your eye up close to the viewing aperture (Figure 111).

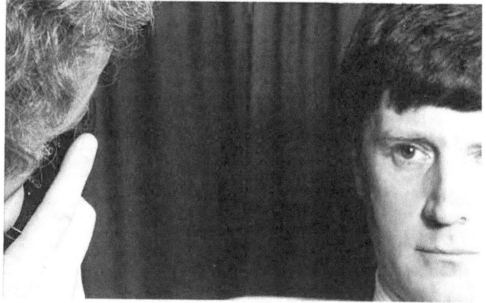

Figure 111

You should see a reddish glow (like the 'red eye' seen in flash photography) through the pupil. This is called the red reflex and is caused by light reflected from the vascular tissue at the back of the eye. Cataracts and some other, more serious, eye problems show up as black opacities within the red reflex. If you see opacities in the red reflex, or no red reflex at all, you should seek advice from an experienced practitioner.

- Keeping the red reflex in view, move yourself and the ophthalmoscope right up close to the eye being examined, moving the focus wheel until the retina comes clearly into view. You should be able to see the blood vessels clearly. Veins look darker than arterioles (Figure 112).

Resist the temptation to move the lens wheel too rapidly when focusing; frantic clicking sounds betray inexperience and small adjustments usually produce the desired clarity. Note that experienced practitioners may start their ophthalmoscopic examination with the +9 (convex) lens selected since this allows them to examine the cornea. They then move the lens selection wheel step by step anticlockwise in order to examine the lens and the vitreous before looking at the retina in detail.

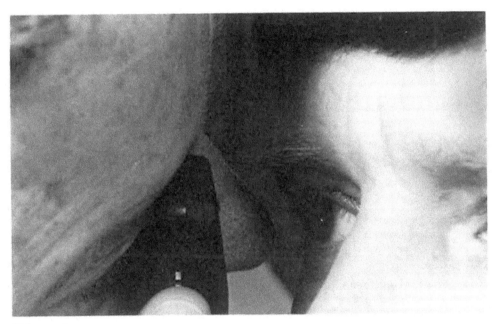

Figure 112

- All blood vessels 'lead to' the optic disc so follow a vessel (probably towards the midline) by moving your head (and thus the ophthalmoscope) a bit until the optic disc comes into view.
- Having studied the outline and form of the optic disc, survey as much as you can of the rest of the retina in a systematic way (e.g. east, north, west, south), either by moving your own head or asking the patient to look inwards, outwards, up and down as you keep the ophthalmoscope more or less still.
- Repeat the examination for the other eye, moving around to the other side of the patient and holding the instrument in the other hand.

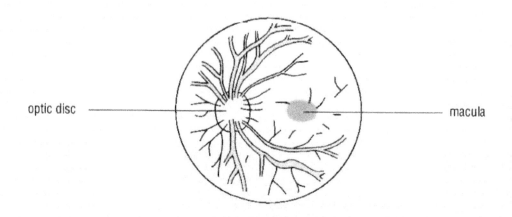

optic disc ———————————————————————— macula

Diagram 3. The normal fundus

What to look for

An experienced ophthalmologist can differentiate a variety of pathologies using a standard ophthalmoscope but, as with all clinical skills, you get good at what you do most often. Complementary practitioners are unlikely to examine fundi on a day-to-day basis and thus should be prepared to seek expert advice whenever something unusual is encountered.

All practitioners should be aware of the retinal damage that may occur in patients with hypertension, diabetes or raised intracranial pressure.

Mild hypertensive 'retinopathy' causes narrowing of the arterioles traversing the retina. As the damage becomes more severe, veins may be seen to be narrowed sharply where they are crossed by arterioles (so called arterio-venous nipping). Very severe damage causes red patchy haemorrhages and white, cotton wool-like 'exudates' to appear. Eventually, papilloedema may be seen (see below).

Diabetic retinopathy consists of a mixture of microaneurysms (small red dots), haemorrhages (larger red blots), hard-looking white exudates, and possibly some soft-looking cotton wool 'exudates'. In severe cases, small, stringy, new blood vessel formation can be seen.

Papilloedema is seen most commonly in patients with severe hypertension or with raised intracranial pressure. The retina looks pinker than normal with dilated veins. The edge of the optic disc looks blurred and indistinct. If seen, the patient should be referred immediately for expert help.

Pictures of these fundoscopic appearances may be found in most standard textbooks of general medicine.

The Auriscope (Otoscope)

These days, auriscopes are usually sold as part of a combined ophthalmoscope/auriscope 'kit' consisting of a handle (containing batteries and on/off rheostat) and interchangeable ophthalmoscope and auriscope heads.

The auriscope attachment usually comes with a number of different sized push-on 'specula' (a speculum is the trumpet-shaped bit that goes in the ear).

The auriscope is simple to use and has no focus wheels or other complex controls. The following hints should help you to obtain a clear view of the external auditory meatus and tympanic membrane.

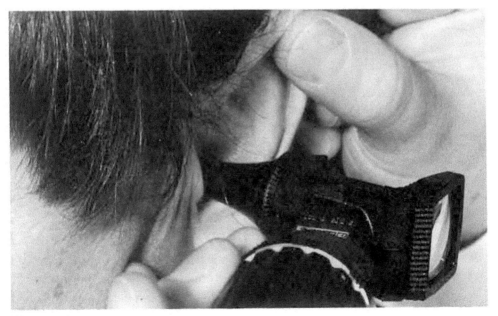

Figure 113

- Always use the largest possible speculum that will fit in the external auditory meatus
- Examine the 'good' ear first
- Do not insert the speculum more than a couple of millimetres into the ear (remember that babies and infants have very short external ear canals and a small speculum inserted just a bit too far could perforate an eardrum)
- Hold the instrument in such a way that a sudden jerk of the patient's head will not cause the speculum to be rammed into their ear (Figure 113)
- With an adult, pulling the auricle upwards, backwards and laterally straightens out the external ear canal and gives a clearer view down to the ear drum
- In babies, pulling the pinna gently downwards and forwards has the same effect
- When looking through the auriscope, try to focus your eye 'into the distance'

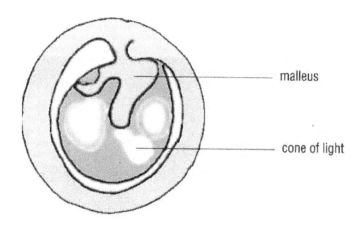

Diagram 4

- Once you have seen a normal, pinkish grey eardrum with its shiny cone of light, you will find it easy to recognize an abnormal or damaged drum
- Practise good hygiene with the specula. Do not put a speculum that has been in an infected ear canal into another ear without adequate sterilization.

3.7 ORTHODOX DIAGNOSTIC TESTS AND LABORATORY REFERENCE VALUES

The clinical diagnostic tests available to the orthodox physician are bewildering both in their number and complexity. You should realize that GPs and hospital doctors often avoid making a definitive diagnosis until the results of the following 'simple' tests are known:

- Urine tests for sugar, protein and infection
- Blood tests for haemoglobin level, red and white cell counts and ESR (erythrocyte sedimentation rate)
- Blood tests for glucose level and also for levels of urea and certain electrolytes such as sodium, potassium and calcium
- Chest x-ray (usually two contrasting views)

These tests are not expensive, not especially invasive (5ml of blood is usually enough) and can answer many diagnostic questions. They are also readily available to almost all practitioners through the numerous laboratories serving the private medical sector. It is important to remember, however, that blood test results by themselves rarely provide a specific diagnosis and laboratories classify their results in terms of 'reference ranges', not 'normality' in an absolute sense. In other words, a patient with a blood test result within the reference range is **likely** to be normal and a result outside the reference range **probably** reflects underlying abnormality. However, reference ranges are the subject of constant review and, in certain cases, debate (e.g. cholesterol). You should therefore guard against drawing conclusions from blood test results unsupported by other clinical data.

Diagnostic tests can be classified under the following specialist hospital department headings:

- Haematology (blood cells and their characteristics)
- Chemical pathology (the chemical composition of the blood)
- Microbiology (detecting the presence of infective agents in blood, sputum, faeces and urine)

147

- Radiography (examining the body with x-rays and ultrasound)
- Nuclear medicine (examining the body with ultra high energy techniques)
- Histopathology (examining biopsy specimens and dead tissues)
- Cardiology (assessing physiological parameters of the CVS)
- Neurology (assessing physiological parameters of the NS)
- Gastro-enterology (examining the inside of the gut using instruments (endoscopes) passed into the GI tract)
- Gynaecology (vaginal examination under anaesthesia, dilatation and curettage, laparoscopy, laparotomy)
- Respiratory medicine (assessing physiological parameters of the RS)
- Urology (examining the internal structure of the UT via x-ray techniques and using endoscopic instruments called cystoscopes)
- Psychology (intelligence and personality testing)

Further information about these and other diagnostic procedures can be found in standard textbooks of medicine and surgery. The following list of laboratory reference values may help you to help your patients interpret the results of any blood or urine tests they may have had. Always check the units of measurement used by the particular laboratory to express test results.

Laboratory Reference Values   Biochemistry

Substance	Reference values
Adrenocorticotrophin (ACTH)	9am: <46 ng/L Midnight: <10 ng/L
Alanine-amino transferase (ALT)	
(Liver function)	Male: 10-50 U/L Female: 5-35 U/L
Albumin	> 15 years old: 35-50 g/L
Aldosterone	100-800 µmol/L
Alkaline phosphatase	
(Liver function/bone disease)	> 15 years old: 30-130 U/L
Aspartate-amino transferase (AST)	
(Liver function)	Male: 0–40 IU/L Female: 0–32 IU/L
Bicarbonate (HCO3)	22 – 29 mmol/L
Bilirubin (Liver function/haemolysis)	0 – 21 µmol/L

Calcitonin	Male: 0–11.8 ng/L Female: 0–4.8 ng/L
Calcium	Adult: 2.2-2.6 mmol/L
Chloride	95–108 mmol/L
Cholesterol	0-5 mmol/L
Cortisol	9am: 137–429 nmol/L
Creatine kinase (CPK)	Male: 40-320 IU/L Female: 25 - 200 IU/L
Creatinine	(Adult) Male: 59-104 μmol/L Female: 45–84 μmo/L
Folate	3.9–26.8 ng/ml
Follicle-stimulating hormone **(FSH)**	Mid-cyle: 4.7–21.5 IU/mL Post-menopausal: 25.8–134.8 IU/mL
Gamma GT (Liver function)	Male: 0-60 IU/L Female: 0-40 IU/L
Glucose (fasting)	<5.5 mmol/L
Iron	5.8–34.5 μmol/L
Lactate dehydrogenase (LOH)	240-480 U/L
Luteinizing hormone (LH) (pre-menopausal)	Follicular phase: 2.4-12.0 IU/mL Mid-cycle: 14.0-95.6 IU/mL Luteal Phase: 1.0-11.4 IU/mL Post-menopausal: 7.7-58.8 IU/mL
Magnesium	0.7–1.0 mmol/L
Parathyroid Hormone (PTH)	10-65 ng/L
Phosphate	Adult: 0.8-1.5 mmol/L
Potassium	Adult: 3.5-5.3 mmol/L
Prolactin	Male: 86–324mU/L Female: 102–496mU/L
Sodium	133-146 mmol/L
Thyroid stimulating hormone (TSH)	0.27–4.2 mU/L
THYROID FUNCTION TESTS FT3	3.1–6.8 pmol/L
FT4	12-22 pmol/L Fasting:
Triglyceride	0–1.7 mmol/L Adult:
Urea	2.5-7.8 mmol/L

Uric acid (urate)	Male: 200–430 μmol/L Female: 140 – 360 μmol/L
Vitamin B12	197–771 ng/L

Key: IU–International Units

Laboratory Reference Values — Haematology

White cell count (WCC)	3.6-11.0 x 10 /L
Red cell count	Male: 4.50-6.50 Female: 3.80-5.80 x10^{12}/L
Haemoglobin	Male: 130-180 g/L Female: 115 - 165 g/L
Haeomocrit (PCV)	Male: 0.40-0.54 L/L Female 0.37-0.47 L/L
Mean cell volume (MCV)	80-100 fL
Mean cell haemoglobin (MCH)	27-32 pg
Neutrophils	1.8-7.5 x 10^9/L
Lymphocytes	1.0-4.0 x 10^9/L
Eosinophils	0.1-0.4 x 10^9/L
Basophils	0.02-0.1 x 10^9/L
Monocytes	0.2-0.8 x 10^9/L
Platelet count	140-400 x 10^9/L
Reticulocyte count	0.2-2.0 %

Erythrocyte sedimentation rate	Male 17-50: 1-7 mm/h
	Male 50+: 2-10 mm/h
	Female 17-50: 3-9 mm/h
	Female 50+: 5-15 mm/
Prothrombin time	h10-14 s
(clotting factors I, II, VII, X)	
Activated partial thromboplastin	23-36 s
time (factors VIII, IX, XI, XII)	

Arterial blood gases reference values

pH: 7.35 to 7.45

PaO$_2$: 10.5 to 14.0 kPa

PaCO$_2$: 4.7 to 6.0 kPa

Note: 1 kPa = 7.6mmHg (atmospheric pressure is about 100 kPa).

Urine Biochemistry Reference Values

Substance	Reference values
Catecholamines	Noradrenaline: 0-500 nmol/24h
	Adrenaline: 0-100 nmol/24h
	Dopamine: 0-3000 nmol/24h
Osmolality	Early morning urine: >600 mmol/Kg
Phosphate (inorganic)	24 hour urine output: 15-50 mmol/24h
Protein	24 hour urine output: 0.00–0.14 g/24h
Sodium	24 hour urine output: 40-220 mmol/24hr

3.8 SAMPLE CASE HISTORY RECORD SHEET

DATE: _____ PRACTITIONER: _____

PRESENTING PROBLEMS / HISTORY OF PRESENTING PROBLEMS

PAST MEDICAL HISTORY

DRUGS

FAMILY HISTORY

SOCIAL HISTORY

Smoking:
Drinking:
Exercise:

DIET

SYSTEMATIC ENQUIRY

Appetite:
Weight:
Bowels:
Urine:
Sleep:
Menstrual:

CLINICAL FINDINGS

Height:
Weight:
Pulse:
BP:

ASSESSMENT

MANAGEMENT PLAN

No. of treatments recommended:

CASE SUMMARY

PROBLEM LIST

Date

Active Problems

Inactive Problems

SURNAME:

FORENAMES:

DOB:

SEX:

DATE OF FIRST CONSULTATION:

ADDRESS:

POSTCODE:

HOME PHONE:

WORK PHONE:

OCCUPATION:

REFERRED BY:

GP NAME:

GP ADDRESS:

GP PHONE:

RESEARCH DATA:

PART FOUR

4.1 SCREENING EXAMINATION OF ALL THE SYSTEMS

With practice, it should be possible to examine any of the systems described in Part 2 in about five minutes each. If you find you are taking significantly longer than this, you are either trying too hard or not practising enough.

However, it is often useful to combine the important elements from all the systems examination procedures into a quick, basic screening examination that can be performed in under 15 minutes.

REMEMBER

- Be kind
- Be gentle but palpate firmly and confidently
- Explain what you are doing
- Try to examine with warm hands
- Do not subject the patient to unnecessary changes of posture
- Be mindful of modesty but remember that examining an area that is not adequately exposed is often worse than not examining it at all
- Hurry slowly
- When interpreting your findings, on the whole trust your first impressions
- Do not sit on the fence

The following sequence is only a suggestion and should be adapted to your own personal style and needs. And remember, when considering the nervous system, some eminent neurologists claim that anyone who can stand on one leg and hop up and down with their eyes closed is unlikely to have a gross neurological abnormality.

- Is the patient well or unwell?
- Alert or drowsy?
- Oriented or disoriented?
- Explain what you are going to do and place the patient in a comfortable position, reclining at 45 degrees

- Examine the hands
- Put thermometer in patient's mouth (if you suspect fever)
- Radial pulses
- Blood pressure
- Read thermometer
- Observe JVP
- Carotid pulses
- Look at face
- Look at conjunctivae and sclerae
- Examine lips, mouth, teeth and fauces (i.e. stick out tongue and say *aaaaaah*)
- Look for swellings in front of neck: ask patient to swallow
- Go behind patient and feel for cervical lymphadenopathy and enlarged thyroid
- Examine breasts (see Part 3.4)
- Examine axillae for lymphadenopathy
- Determine C-S distance and palpate trachea
- Look at chest
- Feel for apex beat
- Feel over praecordium for thrills and heaves
- Listen at the apex with the bell of the stethoscope, with the patient inclined to the left. Listen round into the axilla if you hear a murmur
- Sit the patient forwards and listen with the diaphragm at the left sternal edge (LSE), the aortic area, over the carotids and the pulmonary area. Go back to the LSE and listen for murmurs with the patient holding their breath in expiration
- With the patient still sitting forward, look at the back (noting any spinal deformity) and assess chest expansion and symmetry of movement
- Percuss and auscultate the back of the chest
- Look for sacral oedema
- Lie the patient back and percuss over the clavicles and the front and sides of the chest
- Listen to the front and sides of the chest
- Lie the patient flat and expose the abdomen
- Observe the abdomen
- Looking at the patient's face, feel the abdomen systematically, first superficially then more deeply.
- Feel for enlargement of liver, spleen and kidneys

- Percuss the abdomen
- Listen for bowel sounds with stethoscope
- Feel for femoral pulses
- Look at the inguinal region as patient coughs for evidence of hernia
- Feel for inguinal hernias as patient coughs. If you suspect hernia, you must examine the patient standing
- If patient is male, briefly examine external genitalia
- Sit patient up again to 45 degrees
- Look at the legs
- Assess the leg pulses
- Feel for ankle oedema
- Perform ultra-quick neurological screen as follows:
  Assess leg tone
  Straight leg raising against resistance
  Test knee and ankle jerks
  Plantar responses
  Tuning fork on external malleoli for vibration sense
  Position sense in big toes
  Patient puts arms out in front and closes eyes; look for tremor or drift of one arm
  Ask patient to hold arms steady as you push down on them
  Ask patient to keep eyes closed and put one finger on their nose (each hand)
  Test biceps, triceps and supinator jerks
  Test pupil reactions to light and accommodation
  Look at fundi
  Watch patient walk

Notes

4.2 QUICK REFERENCE

This section summarizes the case history questions and examination routines described in Parts 1 and 2 for use as a quick reference in the clinical situation. The lists of nerve root values for dermatomes, myotomes and tendon reflexes given in Part 2.4 are also included.

History Taking

Personal Details

Presenting Problem

HPP
Onset (time and circumstances)
Progression
Precipitating, aggravating and relieving factors
Associated symptoms
Previous episodes and their management

PMH
Childhood diseases
Illnesses, accidents, hospitalizations, operations
Obstetric history
History of hepatitis/jaundice, rheumatic fever, diabetes, TB, glandular fever, asthma, hay fever, eczema

Drugs
Name, dosage, frequency, length of course, reason prescribed
Painkillers
Sleeping pills
Oral contraceptives
Laxatives/antacids
Vitamins/minerals
Immunizations

Allergies

Notes

FH

Heart disease
Stroke
Diabetes
Other

SH

Smoking habit
Alcohol/recreational drug habit
Exercise
Home situation
Work situation
Hobbies/pastimes

Diet

Systematic enquiry (SQ)

Chest pain
Shortness of breath on exertion
Shortness of breath when lying flat (orthopnoea)
Palpitations
Swelling of the ankles (oedema)
Varicose veins
Cold hands and feet

Catarrh
Earache
Sore throat
Cough/sputum
Coughing up blood (haemoptysis)
Wheeze

Appetite
Weight change
Dental problems
Nausea
Indigestion
Problems swallowing
Vomiting
Abdominal pain
Vomiting blood (haematemesis)
Flatulence
Diarrhoea/constipation

Notes

Unusual looking faeces
Rectal bleeding
Urinary urgency/frequency
Dysuria
Haematuria
Loin pain
Difficulty starting urination
Poor stream
Dribbling/incontinence
Smelly, frothy or discoloured urine

Poor sleep
Headache
Disturbance of vision
Hearing loss
Tinnitus
Dizziness/vertigo
Fainting
Fits
Muscle weakness
Pins and needles
Mood swings
Disturbance of memory/concentration

Heat/cold intolerance
Polyuria/polydipsia

Joint pain/stiffness
Joint swelling
Back ache

Skin rashes
Lumps or bumps
Unusual moles

Sexual problems
Sexually transmitted diseases
Contraception
Infertility
Impotence

Notes

When relevant
Menarche
Cycle length/regularity
Flow
Menstrual pain
Premenstrual disturbance
Bleeding between periods
Vaginal discharge
Painful intercourse
Pregnancies
Miscarriages
Abortions
Contraception
Menopause

Notes

Clinical Examination

The Cardiovascular System
Observe general state
Look at hands
Assess radial pulse
Take BP
Assess JVP
Feel carotid pulses
Assess colour of conjunctivae, tongue and mucous membranes of mouth
Observe then palpate praecordium for apex beat, heaves and thrills
Listen to 'four areas' with diaphragm and bell of stethoscope listening for heart sounds, added sounds and murmurs (some of which are heard more easily with patient in particular position)
Sit patient forward and listen to lung bases for crackles
Check for sacral oedema
Lie patient back, assess peripheral pulses
Assess lower legs for oedema
Look at fundi

Record your findings in the following order:

General observations
Pulse (rate, regularity, character)
Peripheral pulses
BP
JVP/peripheral oedema
Apex beat (position, character)
Thrills/heaves
Heart sounds, added sounds and murmurs

The Respiratory System
Undress patient to waist
Observe general state and chest shape
Look at hands
Turn patient away from you
Observe spine
Palpate for cervical and supraclavicular lymphadenopathy from behind
Assess chest expansion at back
Assess Tactile Vocal Fremitus (upper, middle and lower back and axillae, comparing sides)
Percuss (upper middle and lower back and axillae comparing sides)
Auscultate upper/middle/lower back and axillae (listening for breath sounds and added sounds)

Assess vocal resonance and whispering pectoriloquy if indicated
Turn patient to face you
Assess crico-sternal distance
Palpate position of trachea in suprasternal notch
Palpate apex beat
Assess chest expansion at front
Assess TVF at front
Percuss at front
Auscultate at front

Record your findings in the following order:

General observations (dyspnoea, cyanosis, clubbing, lymphadenopathy)
Respiratory rate
Trachea position and crico-sternal distance
Chest Expansion (Left vs Right)
TVF (Left vs Right)
Percussion note (Left vs Right)
Breath sounds (vesicular or bronchial)/added sounds (wheezes or crackles)

The Gastro-intestinal System
General observation
Look at hands
Look at eyes and in mouth
Lie patient flat with arms by sides and abdomen exposed
Observe abdomen (scars, distension, etc)
Systematic palpation of abdomen, first superficial then deep
Palpate for liver (confirm findings by percussion if necessary)
Palpate for spleen
Palpate for kidneys
Percuss abdomen (assess for shifting dullness if indicated)
Listen for bowel sounds
Examine hernial orifices lying and standing (plus brief look at external genitalia in males)
Consider need for rectal examination

Record your findings in the following order:

General observations
Hands and mouth
Signs of chronic liver disease
Abdomen: softness, tenderness, guarding, rigidity
Masses
Organ enlargement
Bowel sounds

Hernial orifices
(External genitalia)
PR

The Nervous System

Assess consciousness, orientation and memory
Look for tremors and gross weakness of upper limbs
Test co-ordination
Assess function of cranial nerves II to XII:
Visual acuity (II)
Peripheral visual fields (II)
Pupils: symmetry, size and reactions to light and accommodation (II, III)
Eye movements (III, IV, VI)
Nystagmus (cerebellar or vestibular)
Fundi (II)
Trigeminal (V) sensation (including corneal reflex)
Trigeminal (V) motor function (e.g. opening mouth)
Facial nerve (VII) function (muscles of facial expression)
Hearing (VIII), including Weber and Rinne tests
Ask patient to say *aaaaah* – look for symmetrical movement of uvula (IX)
Coughing and swallowing and gag reflex (IX, X)
Ask patient to stick out tongue (XII)
Test strength of sternomastoid and trapezius (XI)

Observe upper limbs for muscle wasting or fasciculation
Assess upper limb tone
Assess upper limb power
Observe lower limbs for muscle wasting or fasciculation
Assess lower limb tone
Assess lower limb power
Elicit tendon jerks and plantar responses
Test vibration sense in feet
Test position sense in feet
Briefly test sensitivity to light touch and pinprick
Perform Romberg test
Watch patient walk

Record your findings in the following order:

Higher functions
Cranial nerves II to XII
Pupils equal size and reacting to light and accommodation (PERLA)
Fundi
Upper limb tone / power / co-ordination
Lower limb tone / power / co-ordination

Reflexes (biceps, supinator, triceps, knee, ankle, plantar) left and right.
Sensory testing (vibration, position sense, light touch, pinprick)

Dermatomes

C4 Tip of shoulder

C5 Lateral aspect of elbow

C6 Thumb

C7 Middle finger

C8 Little finger

T3 Axilla

T8 Costal margin

T10 Umbilicus

T12 Pubis

L3 Knee

L5 Big toe

S1 Little toe

Myotomes

Shoulder abduction:	Deltoid	C5 (axillary nerve)
Elbow flexion:	Biceps	C5/6 (musculocutaneous nerve)
Wrist extension:	Long extensors	C6/7 (radial/post. interosseous n.)
Hand grip:	Intrinsic hand muscles	C8/T1 (ulnar/median nerves)
Hip flexion:	Iliopsoas	L2/3 (femoral nerve)
Knee extension:	Quadriceps	L3/4 (femoral nerve)
Foot dorsiflex:	Tibialis anterior	L4/5 (deep peroneal nerve)
Knee flexion:	Hamstrings	L5/S1 (sciatic nerve)
Foot plantarflex:	Gastrocnemius/Soleus	S1/2 (post. tibial nerve)

Tendon jerks

Biceps C5/6

Supinator C6

Triceps C7/8

Patellar tendon L3/4

Achilles tendon S1/2

Plantar response L5-S2

INDEX